A UNIQUE AND WONDERFUL BOOK, WRITTEN BY AN EXPERT WHO NOT ONLY has extensive experience counselling cancer patients, but also faced multiple recurrences of a life-threatening cancer himself. In addition to this, David is well acquainted with ideas in modern physics, philosophy and consciousness research. It is a platform of understanding, both personal and professional, which sets this book apart from the many texts by professional counsellors and recovered patients published to this point. Maginley fully embraces the perspective, found in nearly all mystical writings and beginning to emerge from modern research, that our essential being is consciousness, not matter. From his broad background he weaves a compelling account of the process of dying as a transition from a limited life in flesh to an expanded awareness of the reality beyond death of the body. He has listened to many stories from people who have temporarily made that transition then returned to tell about it, and he relates his own, extraordinary adventure of this kind.

The sophisticated metaphysical discussions throughout this book are an extremely valuable extension to the usual limited ways in which we attempt to cope with dying, either as afflicted patients or as professionals. However, the emotional impact that permeates this book derives from the great love and compassion David has for his patients. The text is full of moving accounts of people making their own, often fearful steps towards healing or dying, or more often, towards both at once. David has personally followed Campbell's "journey of the hero," stayed here to tell about it, and to support others travelling the same path. It is why I will be recommending the book to all of my cancer patients, and their family members.

— ALASTAIR CUNNINGHAM, O.C., PH.D.
Professor Emeritus of Medical Biophysics, University of Toronto
Author of *The Healing Journey* and *Can the Mind Heal Cancer?*

IN BEYOND SURVIVING: CANCER AND YOUR SPIRITUAL JOURNEY, THIS BRIL-liantly insightful and spirit-nurturing counsellor illumines not only the anxieties of terrible illness, survival, and dying but the challenge of approaching every moment with intention and grace. Facing any life-threatening situation, I want a chaplain like David Maginley at my side.

His book introduces a kaleidoscope of patients — real lives, real surviv-als and real deaths, all interwoven with his own recurring bouts of cancer, his near-death experience and his professional experience as an ordained minister and hospital chaplain. And yet, the book is not so much about him, or even his patients, as it is a reflection on his subject — how we can best approach the reality of chronic, life-threatening suffering and dying. Fundamentally, it is about dealing with the ubiquity of pain and its role as a precipitator of spiritual growth.

The giftedness of his care is evident in every patient interaction and every observation. At his best, Maginley is breathtaking, writing power-ful, deeply true, moving stuff. The result of his multi-faceted background is a uniquely grounded mix of pragmatism and deep spirituality, pro-ducing a book which has the makings of a classic. Highly recommended.

— NANCY EVANS BUSH, MA
President Emeritus of the International Association for Near-Death Studies
Author of *Dancing Past the Dark: Distressing Near-Death Experiences* and
*The Buddha in Hell and Other Alarms: Perspectives on
Distressing Near Death Experiences*

THIS IS A REALLY BEAUTIFUL AND UNIQUE BOOK, FILLED WITH SPIRITUAL insights and obviously a work of love. David Maginley has exquisitely con-veyed the profound role a hospital chaplain plays in patient care, and done so with deep empathy because he's actually been there — on both sides of the veil! Masterfully created, informative, insightful and deeply engaging!

— DR. PENNY SARTORI
Author of *The Wisdom of Near-Death Experiences:
How Understanding NDEs Can Help Us Live More Fully*

BRILLIANT! WISE! COMPASSIONATE! AND SURPRISINGLY FUNNY!! THIS BOOK captures all the attributes and wisdom of a talented and very caring hospital chaplain. David's teachings are simple but powerful — and applicable to anyone at any stage of life's journey. If you want to tap into the body-mind-spirit connection and facilitate healing at the deepest levels in your life, Read This Book.

— DR. ROB RUTLEDGE, MD
Oncologist, Associate Professor, Dalhousie University,
and co-founder of The Healing and Cancer Foundation

BEYOND SURVIVING IS A JOURNEY BEYOND BOUNDARIES. AS A PASTOR, THE words became a part of who I am; guiding me on how to improve my bedside manner, and melting fear of the journey into dying by offering honest conversation and storied experience. The text pushed theological understandings and provided space to ponder the potential of the infinite. It wove together the sacred, as found in many disciplines, and did so grounded in both theology and science. Yet, it remains such an accessible read, filled with grace, that allows for people to consider the journey in finding themselves, God, and life's meaning. I will be sharing this book with colleagues, students, and parishioners, in addition to those facing cancer.

— REV. KIMBER MCNABB
Lutheran Church of the Resurrection

DAVID MAGINLEY PROVIDES INSIGHT INTO THE PEACE AND CLARITY ONE can discover even while facing a cancer diagnosis. His wise and tender words guide the reader to love as the path to a full life here, and an everlasting life beyond. A beautiful reminder that the power to become whole lies within us.

— SHANNON GREEK
Haematology Nurse Practitioner

BEYOND
SURVIVING

BEYOND SURVIVING

CANCER AND YOUR SPIRITUAL JOURNEY

DAVID MAGINLEY

TRISTAN
PRESS

The author of this book does not dispense medical advice or prescribe the use of any technique as a form of treatment for physical or medical issues without the advice of a physician, either directly or indirectly. The intent of the author is only to offer information of a general nature to assist emotional and spiritual well-being. The author and publisher assume no responsibility for your use of the information in this book.

Author's note: All the stories in this book are true and not composites. However, the names and identifying characteristics have been changed for reasons of privacy. Conversations have been related as best the author remembers them.

Cover photo © Freeman Patterson. All rights reserved.
Author Photo: Trevor Allen Photography
Editor: Paula Sarson, PLS Editing Services
Cover and Book Design: Valerie Bellamy, Dog-Ear Book Design,
dog-earbookdesign.com

Scripture quotations are taken from the New Revised Standard Version Bible, copyright 1989, Division of Christian Education of the National Council of the Churches of Christ in the United States of America. Used by permission. All rights reserved.

Tristan Press
PO Box 33131, Quinpool Centre
TRISTAN Halifax, NS B3L 4T6
PRESS Printed in USA

ISBN: 978-0-9958811-1-2

Dedicated to my patients.
Thank you for everything you have taught me.

CONTENTS

Part 4 Near-Death Experiences: The Journey Ends Well

FOREWORD
Freeman Patterson

ALTHOUGH I WAS NOT PRESENT AT THE CONCEPTION OF THIS BOOK, I have been actively involved in evaluating the progress of the pregnancy, and now my friend David Maginley has invited me to participate in the delivery. Thus, my foreword resembles a foresight, because I have knowledge of and a strong feeling for what you, the reader, are about to experience. Through this book and the personal stories it contains you will explore the experience of cancer holistically.

Cancer always occurs within a specific situation. It affects — physically, emotionally, and spiritually — not just the person who has received the diagnosis, but everybody who shares their life. Cancer is a trip in all three dimensions simultaneously, a short- or long-term adventure that holds the dark potential for unnecessary forms of suffering and grief while offering an unparalleled opportunity for major personal growth and spiritual development. David knows these possibilities intimately, both because he has grappled with four occurrences of cancer himself and because he is at the working face of cancer at a major hospital every day of his professional life.

David lives with cancer, but he always looks beyond survival to the fullness of life — regardless of whether a patient will survive the illness. He considers it a privilege to share this time when questions of meaning become central to a patient, family, and friends and to encourage and help them examine and transcend their fears of suffering, loss, death, and the afterlife. David avoids nothing; he does not beat around the bush. He tells it like it is.

If you have experienced cancer personally, if you have lived with or cared for somebody with cancer, if you have suffered the loss of somebody you loved deeply, if you worry about developing cancer yourself, or if you keenly desire spiritual growth, you will find in these pages the knowledge, understanding, profound caring, and deep love that will provide you with hope, guidance, sustenance, and peace.

Anticipate a compelling read!

PREFACE

I STOOD BY HER BODY, TRYING TO DISCERN IF THE SPIRIT THAT HAD animated it was still hovering in the room, watching us. An elderly woman of great character, she had been the anchor of her family even as cancer reduced her to a wisp of what was. The monitors and instruments that measured life were mute. They never could detect her consciousness anyway, only the effects of its presence — the rise and fall of breath, the rhythms of heart and brain. But what of her mind? What of her essence? As her family wept at the bedside, I glanced at a corner of the ceiling, certain that she continued — because I remembered that I had, when I died.

For over fifteen years, I have been a spiritual counselor at a major cancer center. I've sat with hundreds as they've fought for more moments of life, and hundreds during that last, precious moment. I can appreciate both perspectives not only as a chaplain, but also as a four-time cancer survivor. This gives me unique insight into my patients' experience, an intensified empathy to support them in the crisis of their lives, and to learn from them what is most important in this one — to love deeply, to be real, to know that life has purpose, and to make a difference by living it. These are the lessons cancer brings to us. This is the homework, and it is unavoidable.

I wrote this book to help with that homework, to be intentional about the growth that can come through cancer, to find hope and deep meaning in what initially is fear and chaos. There's more to engaging spirituality than prayer or faith. Wrapped up in that ephemeral awareness is the hard work of harnessing the wisdom of grief, love, and mortality to amplify life and the connection to our immortal nature. There is robust (though often dismissed) evidence showing how that immortal nature is indeed very real. Tapping into it enables us to move beyond surviving cancer to transforming our conscious selves so that we resonate with the Divine. And, as you may be hoping, it can also improve our prognosis and our experience of life.

Engaging the spiritual dimension of cancer means more than asking the proverbial question, "Why me." That's a great place to start, but we need to go further, for behind that question is a host of powerful, vulnerable emotions: how everything suddenly feels fragile, how it all could fall apart, how overwhelmed we are. When life is no longer comfortable and secure, love becomes our greatest struggle as well as our greatest strength. The heart breaks just thinking about telling family of the diagnosis, yet rallies for their sake to face what may lie ahead. Even with a treatable cancer, people ask in the silence of their hearts, "What if I don't make it? If I die, will I continue on in some way? Will I still be connected to those I love?" These are the questions forced on us when hit with a crisis that will strike over 40 percent of North Americans.[1] Though survival rates are improving, the disease and that word "cancer" still hold tremendous power. Whatever the prognosis, cancer will cause us to contemplate life and, if we do our homework, deepen our love. We can do more than go through cancer; we can grow through cancer. We can touch on our true significance, even while feeling small and frail. I hope this book supports you in that endeavor, transforming your world by transforming your experience of it.

If you have cancer, are supporting one who does, or have lost someone to this epidemic disease, there can be no greater gift than uncovering, through love, the astonishing miracle of who you truly are: an immortal, beautiful, unique expression of God. I confidently say this because I frequently hear of mystical experiences; a spiritual apparition, profound peace and light, even a glimpse of heaven. Regardless of the outcome — whether you live or die — these moments, more than any other, show that while we battle against cancer with every ounce of strength, it is just as important to see death not as a failure, but a transformation — one we stave off as long as possible — but when it comes, how wonderful to find it does not destroy us!

We will explore all this through four sections. Part 1 reviews the realities of cancer, what it's like to receive a diagnosis, and treatment options currently available. The crisis leads to questions of meaning and hope. These are spiritual issues, for they address who we are independent of the body, if and how we matter in the big picture.

Part 2 explores core lessons in the spiritual homework thrust upon us by cancer: forgiveness and grief. All souls are wounded. Cancer is a powerful impetus to address the difficult work of reconciliation, sorrow, and partnering with our mind in such a way as to cultivate a stronger and more compassionate presence. And then there are the miracles — those remarkable survivors who defy the odds. The role spirituality plays in this cannot be overstated, and while it does not guarantee victory, it does enable something even greater: a deeper, more authentic character — one that not only shines in this world, but also manifests light from the next.

Part 3 examines the nature of our immortal self: the soul. It begins by wrestling with the age-old mystery of consciousness. What is the nature of mind? What animates us and produces self-awareness? One perspective sees consciousness as an emergent property of the brain; the other sees consciousness as mediated through it. This is a subtle but significant difference, for the second perspective concludes that material reality, everything we call "real," arises from consciousness. It points to the spiritual foundation for all that is.

Exploring the link between spirit and flesh may sound esoteric, but it is more accessible than you may think, for just as we have a physical anatomy, we also have a spiritual or energetic anatomy. As a cancer patient, it's exciting to consider that you are more than your body, more than your brain, and are connected to a healing realm beyond this one. While the nature of that reality cannot be understood with the tools of this one, quantum physics gives us a tantalizing glimpse as to how thin the veil between these worlds may be.

Part 4 examines the most exciting part of that journey: that it continues long after our bodies do not. Near-death experiences (NDEs), a phenomenon reported throughout time and cultures, give us a glimpse of what awaits us. They also reveal the underlying agenda of life: to evolve through love so we can then continue on the spiritual journey. The characteristics of NDEs are explored, along with the difficulty we have in accepting them.

The term "consciousness" is central to our explorations, and will be used in reference both to our individual selves and to the spiritual level of reality that sustains this one. How odd that the experience we take for granted — being alive and aware, is actually the greatest mystery to science. In fact, the contemporary struggle between science and faith is not a matter of the existence of God, but of the nature of consciousness. This term is a worthy successor for the more misunderstood term "soul" that connotes duality — I have a soul — something opposed to the body, somehow superior and separate. It also implies an artificial barrier between this world and the next, a barrier that is more permeable than we realize, for whether you are alive or dead, you *are* a consciousness.

All of this will be presented through the weave of my own cancer journey, the journeys of my patients, and reflections on hope, courage, and continued existence beyond this realm. We will not do this lightly. You will find no simple encouragements here to support your comfort. It is an extremely dangerous journey we are on, one in which temporarily losing faith may actually be a requirement in developing a more robust and supportive connection to something greater. Solitude and a sense of abandonment are fertile, frightening fields to cross, especially when we carry so much with us into the wilderness. Cancer throws everyone into that landscape, ripping the carpet of security out from underneath. Suddenly everything is different, and the next breath can feel like such a gift. How does one make this journey?

Imagine (or remember) receiving a cancer diagnosis. Even when surrounded by love, suddenly you feel overwhelmed and afraid. So, you rally yourself, committing body, mind, and soul to the task of beating this disease. Beyond changes to diet and exercise, you place your body into the hands of the medical team. At times your greatest adversary is your own mind, which you wrestle with as you negotiate the ups and downs of hope and worry.

As for the spirit, well, you pray. Is there anything else? Maybe you go to church, but that rarely helps if it's not part of your faith practice already. Maybe you explore meditation or yoga, or pick up a book by a life coach or cancer survivor. Now, here you sit, holding another. Let this be a guide, of sorts, through the wilderness of cancer. Above all, I hope it will support you in your growth, and bring home the promise that you are so much more than flesh and blood. And I hope that it will do so with intelligence, respect, and awe.

Never could I have imagined I would deal with life-threatening tumors four times, that cancer would bring me repeatedly to the edge of death, or that I would slip over that edge and return; an experience so infused with love, belonging, awareness, and joy that those who've had it are forever changed. Never would I have imagined that my ministry would lead me beyond the borders of conventional faith to study the nature of consciousness, to learn from the dying what it is to live, or to discover that to love is nothing less than spiritual evolution in action. Perhaps you, too, cannot imagine what the road of cancer will bring. I invite you to walk it as part of your spiritual journey. Go beyond surviving cancer — use it to fuel your growth, expand your consciousness, heal your heart, and transform your life.

BEYOND SURVIVING

Cancer and Your Spiritual Journey

PART 1

REALITIES OF CANCER:
THE JOURNEY IS DANGEROUS

FIRST TUMOR

Don't waste a crisis.

— MYRON F. WEINER, MD

THERE WAS SO MUCH BLOOD, BUT SURPRISINGLY NO PAIN. THE SHOCK-ing stream was thick and dark. I stared at it in confusion. Had something happened in my sleep? Did I suffer an injury? My skin showed no bruising, my body felt no trauma. Yet the pleasant, private, universal morning ritual of urination had suddenly become a freakish horror show. Realizing I would soon lose consciousness, I pulled up my pants and went in search of my mother.

Chromatic scales stumbled with me down the hall as I approached the music room; the student wrestling with Bach reminded me it was Saturday morning. My mother would be teaching piano until late in the day, and he would be among a steady stream of pupils flowing through the house until supper. Knowing my own crisis would have to derail that routine, I still hesitated at the door. At seventeen, interrupting a lesson felt as awkward as it did when I was a little boy. But while my mind was clogged with apprehension, my bladder was filling with blood, so I leaned in and quietly asked Mom to step into the kitchen.

"Oh, good morning, David. How was your night?"

"Something's up. Could I speak with you for a moment?" I feigned a smile so as not to distress her with my impending collapse.

"What is it? I won't be long here. Why don't you get some breakfast, and put on the coffee, too." Then, turning to her student, "Join us on the deck by the pool. It's such a lovely morning." Our home had always had a revolving door, and my mother thrived on company and conversation.

"No," I said. "I'd really like a word with you." She was beginning to look blurry.

"Hold on. Ali, run over this line a few more times. What is it, David?" She still wasn't moving from the room.

I leaned in and whispered, "I'm bleeding and am about to collapse."

There was a pause, a look of confusion. "What do you mean?"

"I need to get to a hospital. Right now."

Her eyes shot wide open. "Oh, God! Oh no!" She began to look for blood on my body.

"No, Mom, I'm holding it in. But we should really get going."

With urgent yet deft politeness, she turned to her student and asked his opinion! I later learned that he was not only one of her advanced pupils, but also the son of a physician, and studying medicine himself. After I awkwardly explained how I was hemorrhaging, he firmly agreed, "You should go to emergency."

With the commanding force only a mother can produce to summon the troops, she shifted gears. "Robin, we're going to the hospital!"

My stepfather bellowed back from the upstairs bathroom, his voice like a cackling crow, squawking a prolonged "Whaaaat?" through toothpaste and morning delirium. It took him hours to prepare for a leisurely day.

"Oh, God. I can't wait for him," she muttered. "We're going to the hospital! Get everyone up!" There were five other siblings and stepsiblings to pull into consciousness and clothing. That could take forever. I supposed I had about a minute left.

"No, no, Mom, let's just go, you and me. Now. Please."

Again the student urged, "Just go!"

I put on my jacket and headed to the car. She drove. Fast. In the wrong direction! I realized the clinic was closer, a few blocks away, and decided that must be where she's headed. Would it even be open? Fortunately, the door swung easily and the receptionist was just as bright and friendly as the Saskatchewan sunshine.

"Good morning! Beautiful out there, isn't it?"

Mom came at the desk with restrained panic. "My son's bleeding," she said, peeling the edge off the counter as she smiled. "We need a doctor."

The receptionist looked at me for a wound, a stain. I smiled awkwardly. "Hi."

"This really is an emergency." Mom's eyes were a bit crazed. I moved to the chair. A nurse appeared and took me to one of the clinic rooms, where I sat on the narrow examination bed and tried to look normal. I unconsciously fixed my bedhead as she smiled and chatted through her initial assessment. Even though I was an anxious, awkward, and, at the moment, ashen youth, I recall thinking how cute she was (the seventeen-year-old male mind is a ridiculous apparatus), and then feeling embarrassed as I realized an examination would soon follow. There are times a young man should keep his blood pressure where it belongs.

Fortunately, she simply asked for a sample, then took it to the doctor. I waited. Looked around. Anatomical posters showing polyps and tumors are not comforting. Interesting, yes. Especially the three-dimensional ones, where you can feel the bumps and curves, and imagine them growing and bleeding into your bladder. Posters of mountain meadows would be much better — something comforting and beautiful, something to calm a patient. I played with a stethoscope, put it to my heart to hear if it had much juice left, and contemplated the possibilities. Perhaps a stream of blood mixed with urine was actually something quite minor. Just a nick. Could be nothing, really. And I wasn't unconscious yet. Maybe this will just need a bandage.

Then a different nurse arrived, a huge nurse. "OK, young man, drop the pants." She stood blocking the light from the hallway as she made the decree, clearly on a mission with a massive needle.

"Excuse me?"

"Now, don't be nervous, this won't hurt a bit. Just turn around and place your hands on the bed."

This didn't make sense. "I don't want that," I stammered. "I don't understand." She approached with obvious experience in dealing with difficult subjects. With a firm hand and quick aim, she gave me little time to think. My pants were halfway down before I knew it. "Now, now, it won't feel bad, just a quick prick."

I reached out my arm in protest. "I really don't want that. I feel better. I think I can go home now."

She would have nothing of it, and had me bent over like a rodeo calf in one move.

Then the door burst open. "What are you doing?" The doctor looked at the nurse with shock. "That's for the patient in the next room!"

My savior! My liberator! My goodness, my pants were still down! Awkwardly, I pulled them up and slumped on the bench. The assailant quickly left the room.

"I'm sorry, David," the doctor said. "That needle would have knocked you flat on the floor. It's a good thing you held her off." Her smile was both abashed and comforting.

"Aw, wasn't so bad," I lied. "I can take care of myself." She was gracious enough not to allow me further embarrassment, and turned to a container of blood. My blood.

"You're definitely bleeding inside, but it's not dangerous. I want to do a quick examination and send you to the hospital for further tests."

"Examination?" Modesty and nerves clouded my teenage mind. "I don't have to pull down my pants again, do I?"

"No," she laughed. "Just relax."

Blood pressure was low. Odd, given my ordeal. Unless I didn't have much left. After a few routine questions, we were on our way. I had a feeling Mom was not going to get back to her students any time soon. And I wasn't going to get breakfast, in case they needed to do scans. My gut was in knots as I realized the day was only going to get worse. I can't think well on an empty stomach, on top of a medical crisis and medication mistakes. We would soon find out that nurse was the least of my problems.

HOSPITALS ARE STRESSFUL PLACES, AND IT BEGINS IN THE PARKING LOT. One always tries to find a spot close to the entrance, tries to find a wheelchair, tries to keep calm while waiting in line, waiting in the receiving room, waiting in the examination room.... That's why they call us patients — subliminal compliance.

Dr. Afridi arrived, a warm and positive man with a surprising ability to instill confidence and calm with just his tone, all the while wasting no time with chit-chat. There would be no talk of the weather with this guy. I liked him right away. Which is a good thing — you place your life in the hands of the doctor, relying on expertise that can only be wrought through years of training and decades of experience. Then, all that confidence is swallowed up in anxiety as he explains what he's going to do.

"I'm going to perform a cystoscopy. Basically, lay you back and insert a scope about the thickness of a pencil up your penis, and look in your bladder."

Suddenly, the world looked fuzzy again. I calculated how far the door was from the chair.

Dr. Afridi continued, "The scope is inserted into your urethra. If it has a spot that's too narrow, I can insert other smaller instruments to gradually enlarge the opening. Surgical devices can also be inserted through the scope to take tissue samples from your bladder. I'll be able to see what's causing this bleeding, and take a biopsy. It will just be a little uncomfortable."

"You mean I'll be awake?"

"Yes, but I'll use some freezing, so you shouldn't feel much."

Freezing. My penis. With a needle. Where's that door? But before I could make my move, a nurse took me to the change room, where I found a miniskirt and a pair of feminine pads to wear on my feet. I should explain:

I am a beanpole, all the more when I was seventeen. At six foot eight, I struggle to fit in this world, let alone a hospital gown, which barely covers my dignity. My height has always been a bother, and I've never used it to my advantage.

First day of high school the basketball coach, an oddly short, rotund, and hairy man, simply said to me, "You're going to play, right?" I apologized, and answered, no, I was not going to play. I had the coordination of a newborn giraffe. Little did I know if I had said yes that man could have transformed awkwardness into agility, shyness into confidence. Instead, I tried for most of my life to blend in, stand at the back, slouch. How very odd that God had opposite plans for me, that I would one day be ordained and stand week after week in front of so many people.

On this day, though, I had a long way to go in growing into my body, and even further to grow into someone I could never imagine — someone who could not only tolerate a needle, but stand compassionately in the presence of pain and death, and not lose hope or consciousness. I'm deeply grateful for that growth. As for my body's growth, well, I still can't dunk it.

In the change room, I tore the sponge slippers on my size 13 feet, tugged the hospital gown over my lap, crossed my legs, and looked around nervously for a blanket. The porter soon arrived to take me to the procedure room. I had to empty my bladder before the procedure and was relieved to find I had nothing to empty. No urine. No blood. No problem! I'm healed! It's a miracle! They didn't buy it.

"Lie back on the table," the nurse instructed. (I don't fit.) "Place your feet up on the stirrups." Suddenly, I was filled with an overwhelming vulnerability. Breath became short, sweat broke out on my forehead. I wanted to run.

Dr. Afridi entered, gowned in green, and said the most ridiculous thing: "Relax, David. It's going to be fine." I didn't realize I was shaking with rigors.

"Oh, I'm OK," I said through chattering teeth.

"This won't take long. I'm going to freeze the area. It may feel a bit cold." The "area." Surely it must be the size of a pea by now.

I felt something cold, some pressure. My head started to spin. "Ah, I don't feel so good," I mumbled as my head flopped to the side. I was as pale as a ghost.

"Hang in there, David." The nurse put a cold compress on my head. The room was tilting at a strange angle. My bladder felt cold and full — saline pumped in to inflate it for the examination.

Then Dr. Afridi said the most wonderful word: "Done!" I breathed deep, head still spinning. "You did just fine. It's over. Get yourself dressed, and I'll see you in my office." And with that, I carefully rose, had some orange juice, and staggered to my clothes, to my mother, and to the news of what had turned a summer Saturday morning on its head.

"How are you, sweetie? Not looking so hot."

I slumped in the seat next to her, and put my head between my knees.

Dr. Afridi didn't take long to return. The news wasn't good. "You have a tumor, about the size of an almond, hanging in the dome of your bladder," he explained. "It's very vascular, and lucky for you, started bleeding, so I was able to find it. We have to take it out. It's going to mean an operation, and a stay in the hospital. Now, there are a few options — you have a choice in how extensive the surgery can be. First choice: I can remove the tumor through another cystoscopy, but I don't get to see how it's affecting the tissue around it. Second: I can remove the dome of your bladder with the tumor — that's going to mean an incision in your belly and a longer stay in hospital. If it's malignant, that would be the best choice, the one I recommend. We want to remove the cells associated with it, not just the tumor. The third choice: if you want to eliminate all risk of future recurrence, remove your bladder. This would mean having a bag on the outside of your body to urinate into. This would also mean you would be impotent, unable to have an erection. We would look at a penile implant in that case, but you wouldn't be able to have children any time in the future. Given your young age, I would advise against that one, but it does ensure your best prognosis."

Suddenly, things had become a lot more serious than I ever anticipated. Anyone who has received a cancer diagnosis knows the delay that occurs between hearing the doctor say the words and you comprehending them.

It's called "cognitive dissonance" — the mental stress experienced when your reality is shattered by another one, such as "I'm healthy and will live to a ripe old age," compared to, "I have cancer and could die." A circuit breaker flips in your mind. This is actually a form of shock, marked by dizziness, dread, guilt, anger, embarrassment, or anxiety, but the most common response is to tune out. You can't hear anything, can't understand, even the conversation you're currently having turns into a kind of background hum, a numbing, murky fog through which you continue smiling, nodding, acting as if you're all there when you're anything but. This new reality is incompatible with yours, so one of them will have to be rejected for a while, giving you time to adjust. Grieve. Wail and kick and scream and cram in a mid-life crisis or some really intense retail therapy. Do an instantaneous life review, then go on a binge because it really wasn't anything you thought it would be. This is what I wanted to do: condense a lifetime into whatever I had left.

So, though I weighed the options and decided on the second choice — remove the dome of my bladder — nonetheless, I was actively blocking the reality of cancer. I knew I had a tumor, but being seventeen and suddenly stunned, I did not realize what that implied. And I did not want to know. Nor could I imagine how this experience would change my life. Yet in only a few days a new perspective emerged, an engagement with life that led me out of timidity and thrust me into mindful awareness of how precious and fleeting each moment is. I did not want to miss any more of them because of meekness. In fact, I developed a motto, a creed of sorts: "Live fast, love hard, leave clean underwear." It was not an excuse for recklessness. Rather, it was a philosophy of *carpe diem*: take risks, experience life with appreciation and gratitude, and don't leave a mess behind you when you leave. It was the perfect expression of a teenage mind, but it never led me to do anything risky or disrespectful. I simply wanted to dive in and become the hero of my own life, however brief that life may be.

As I lay on the surgical table weeks later, I reflected on that life. Breathing in the anesthetic and plummeting to unconsciousness, I prayed I would have time to live it well.

THE FOG OF ANESTHETIC INDUCED A DREAM-LIKE BORDERLAND: I COULD hear what others were saying, but could not respond. The bed tilted oddly as I moved my head. The room swam.

"David, it's the nurse. You've had an operation. You're in recovery. Can you open your eyes?"

No, no. Go away, I thought. What are you doing in my bedroom?

"Open your eyes, David. Tell me your name. Do you know where you are?"

I moaned. I growled. I began to surface. Didn't I just close my eyes a minute ago? I wondered. Oh, my head feels heavy. Then I remembered: operation, cancer, hospital. Dr. Afridi removed the tumor in my bladder. Two weeks before it had been hemorrhaging, and now it was in the pathology lab. Soon I would find out how bad things really were.

I opened one eye. Her face was fuzzy. Shadows moved behind yellow curtains. The room was large and smelled faintly sweet and clean. She smiled.

"There you are. We'll be taking you up to your room shortly. Just rest awhile and the porter will come and get you."

You're very kind. Please go away, I thought.

The bed was moving. Left, right, forward … now up — an elevator. I rolled to my side; finally still in my hospital room. I felt the weight of warm blankets and dreamed of summer days, unaware of the chair being pulled up by my side.

"I want to know everything."

"About what, sweetie?" my mother asked.

"About everything."

Recovery was a special time marked by awakened gratitude. Nurses going about their daily tasks were angels in my eyes, especially one who came into my room, pulled the curtains to the side, gave me a wink, and said, "Good morning, sunshine!" Oh, so impressionable.

I savored her smile with a secret crush, until one day I heard her walk into another patient's room, pull the curtains, and say, "Good morning, sunshine!" After momentary heartache, I realized that if she made all the patients feel the way she made me feel, then she was a truly special person. Maturity inches forward through such insights.

The tumor proved to be a fascinating anomaly called paraganglioma.

"Over 95 percent of these are benign," Dr. Afridi said with a reassuring smile. "You're a very lucky young man. And I think you chose the best surgical option. I removed the dome of your bladder, which was clear, so there's no spread, and you can go on with a normal life. We'll take the stitches out in a couple of weeks. Until then, let your mother take care of you and don't lift anything heavier than a glass of water."

Mom smiled, squeezing my hand. "That's wonderful," she said. "Wonderful! Thank you, doctor."

She bought him a bottle of wine and some wind chimes, and he was forever the hero for saving her son. Over the decades ahead, it seemed he did not forget me, which evoked profound admiration that I stumbled to express. He was an amazing man, and I felt like his only patient.

WEEKS LATER, MY FINGERS TRACED THE SCAR ON MY STOMACH AS I GAZED at the textbook in the medical library. "Paraganglioma: a neuroendocrine neoplasm … 97% are benign and cured by surgical removal; the remaining 3% are malignant because they are able to produce distant metastases."[2] I had some deciphering to do. Neuroendocrine: arising from the hormonal system. Neoplasm: a tumor. Benign: not cancer … not cancer. The rest didn't matter. I closed the book, breathed in the musty aroma that rose from its pages, and walked into the sunshine.

I felt like I had dodged a bullet. I thought I was among the lucky ones. Never could I have imagined there would be more tumors. It would take years to realize they were actually malignant. For most cancers, this is determined quickly by analyzing the histology, or structure of the tumor cells, but in my case it would be revealed by their behavior; they spread slowly to distant tissues (metastasized). They threaten life not by taking over the body, but by their metabolic activity — these things were time-bombs, packed with enough adrenaline to cause instant death. They may be the single most high-risk tumors physicians treat.[3]

Unaware of the dangers ahead, I was instead filled with a new resolve to live life well, and a newfound curiosity for what life was about. That summer, I enrolled at the University of Saskatchewan, and dove into philosophy and world religions. It was a ridiculous career move — I never wanted to teach and didn't consider myself an academic. What could I do with such a degree? I didn't care; I just wanted to explore the meaning of life. I chose this path with no recollection of the conversation with my mother at the bedside, and I've had no memory, to this day, of that exchange. When I told her of my decision, she simply smiled.

CHAPTER 2

DIAGNOSIS AND TREATMENT

We must embrace pain and burn it as fuel for our journey.
— KENJI MIYAZAWA

THE SHOCK

CANCER. THE WORD AMPLIFIES OUR FRAILTY, AWAKENS OUR MOR-tality, and activates the existential crisis that can either stir us with vitality or plunge us into despair. Some people appear to receive their diagnosis with a calm demeanor. They play it cool and ask intelligent questions. They review treatment options, check their calendar to see how it will affect their schedule, without realizing how that schedule could be upset for years. Then there are those who break down and sob right away, crumbling into their partner's arms.

It's the first ones I worry about. They will walk from the doctor's office, and before they've stepped into their car, the details will begin to blur. Amnesia will set in. The mind will blank out the bulk of the conversation, even of the diagnosis itself. Here's that cognitive dissonance, the mental stress experienced when your reality is shattered by another. It's certainly not exclusive to cancer — it can be triggered by exposure to any ideas, beliefs, values, or emotions that are so troubling they cause you to tune out. How critical, then, to have a wingman, a second set of ears in the doctor's office. They can hear the news without the filters automatically kicking in. Now, those filters are not necessarily bad. They are part of the fight-or-flight mechanism wired into every living creature, developed over millions of years of evolution. Cognitive dissonance can actually ensure your emotional survival. By blanking out, going into shock, you are able to function (sometimes in the most rudimentary ways) and make yourself do what needs to be done, whether that be making a meal or having a bone marrow biopsy. We adapt gradually to this new reality through the course of treatment, and beyond.

Some have said that it was not until chemotherapy was dripping into their body that it truly hit them: I have cancer. I have cancer. The sentence becomes a dark mantra, hypnotic and bleak. Others realize it when the treatments are over. Isn't that the point one is supposed to be happy, relieved, and jubilant for making it through? Instead, there is a melancholy period, a no-man's land between illness and health. You do not feel the congratulations given by friends and family. You are not able to get on with your life. You do not feel safe. Instead, you feel fatigued, restless, and uncertain. Treatment side effects may handicap your days, while in the dark of night, realization dawns of what you have endured. This emotional homework can continue for years as you slowly integrate the experience of cancer and struggle to find a new normal. You even resist claiming the title of "survivor." With cancer in the shadows and "normal" long gone, that trophy just doesn't feel yours to own. Many simply say they were lucky.

There are those who quickly realize the stakes, then run far ahead of the diagnosis. Even though many cancers are treatable and some very common ones curable, they hear only one word: tumor. For them, tumor means cancer, and cancer means death. So, instead of blanking out they go into fight mode. The to-do list suddenly becomes very full, and they feel like there's not much time left to complete it. I've found that men in particular will become busy fixing up the homestead, tidying the yard, tackling the backlog at work — essentially packing for the final trip in an effort to leave everything in order for their loved ones. This is an effective tool in distraction, and while it's avoiding the emotional homework, it certainly gets the house clean.

Eventually, it seeps in, that little voice, saying over and over, "I have cancer. I could die." This is a secret world within many patients. From the moment of diagnosis, you negotiate with mortality, thinking of the milestones you want to reach, wondering what you have to do to get there: to see your children grow, to have them marry, to be blessed with grandchildren, to pay off the house. And then you look at your wife, your kids, your mother ... your toast and tea, warm in your hands. Nothing looks the same. Everything is fleeting, fragile, and so precious. In that moment of realization your heart breaks open, tears well up, and you know what you dare not say to your loved ones: this could be the end.

WHAT IS CANCER?

CANCER IS A FOREIGN LAND TO THOSE WHO ARE DIAGNOSED. ALTHOUGH this book is mainly about the spiritual dimensions of cancer, we can discuss them only when we have a good foundation in the fundamentals of cancer and treatment options. Then we can consider what role spirituality plays in the journey.

Cancer is not a disease. It is a disease process: cells growing out of control. Breast cancer is breast cells growing where they should not. Colon cancer is colon cells growing where they should not. There are, in fact, over two hundred types of cancer, caused by both external factors (such as tobacco, chemicals, and radiation) and internal factors (such as mutations, hormones, immune conditions). Together, breast, lung, prostate, and colorectal cancer make up more than half of all cancers diagnosed each year.[4,5] Ten or more years often pass between exposure to external factors and detectable cancer. How these factors influence the development of cancer is in many ways a mystery. An even greater puzzle is how we might influence disease by our thoughts and feelings. This area is largely dismissed in cancer research, but new understandings of the mind-body connection are compelling us to consider that we can affect cancer with consciousness itself. We'll explore that later in the book.

Cancer has a range of severity. For instance, skin cancer (melanoma) caught early is highly treatable and prognosis is very good for a long and full life. Pancreatic cancer is more aggressive, and even when caught early, can be life-threatening. Yet, even a person who has had uterine cysts removed (precancerous cells, very treatable and not life-threatening) may reflect briefly on death because of that word "cancer" (even though it has "pre-" in front of it, meaning that if left alone, the cells could develop into cancer).

When people think of cancer, they inevitably conceive of the emaciated figure in a hospital bed, wracked by nausea, vomiting, diarrhea, and pain. While this can be the case in advanced stages for some cancers, most patients look like any average, healthy individual. This is in contrast to how they may feel walking around with the disease. "You look great!" can become an encouragement that crushes connection to the reality within.

Cancer Treatments

CANCER IS TREATED IN A VARIETY OF WAYS: SURGERY, CHEMOTHERAPY, radiation, hormone therapy, biological therapy, and targeted therapy. Sometimes these are used in combination, and always they are being refined and advanced. It's actually a very exciting and hopeful time in the history of cancer care. Exponential advancements in computer intelligence and genetics place us on the edge of staggering breakthroughs we will see in our lifetime. I'm very hopeful that the standard treatments currently available, while they might not provide a cure, may provide time until one comes.

Surgery is what saved me. It's used for the removal of isolated tumors and those that have begun to spread (metastases). It can involve everything from a minor biopsy done with scopes that require only a small incision, to massive operations like a Sugarbaker procedure, in which the intestines are lifted from the abdominal cavity, which is then washed in heated chemotherapy to destroy any hidden cancer cells. Sometimes the cancer is found to be too extensive, in which case the patient is closed and must consider palliative care or alternative therapies.

Chemotherapy is the use of chemicals to destroy cancer. It can be one drug or a mixture of drugs, administered by pills or intravenously. Many associate chemo with poison, which, in fact, it is. But these are poisons specifically targeted for certain conditions, administered in the optimal dose that will be most toxic to the disease, but tolerable for the body. Because cancer can be so aggressive, chemotherapy is often given at the maximum dose first, while the body is strong enough to withstand it, then subsequent doses are reduced (titrated) as the body becomes weaker.

Chemotherapy is given on both an inpatient and outpatient basis, depending on the type needed, the condition of the patient, and the time required to recover from each dose. It is often given in cycles. One cycle is generally the amount of chemo you receive in a month, and overall treatment can vary from weeks, months, and in a few cases, years. If a scan shows the cancer has disappeared, chemo may continue for one to two cycles to eradicate all microscopic remains. If the cancer shrinks but does not disappear, chemotherapy may be continued as long as it can be tolerated. If the cancer grows, chemo may be stopped.

Some cancers, like lymphoma or leukemia, can take over the immune system by growing in the bone marrow, where blood is made. The plan may then be to have a **bone marrow transplant**, in which the diseased marrow is destroyed through chemo, then replaced with healthy stem cells. This is also called a blood marrow or a stem cell transplant. As I write this, there are three kinds of transplants, but given the rate of developments, in as little as five years there could be something that replaces transplants altogether.

The first kind is autologous, in which your own stem cells are collected, and then your immune system is wiped out through heavy chemotherapy. Your banked stem cells are then reintroduced to your body, to set up shop in the bone marrow, and hopefully, get to work producing entirely new blood components: platelets, red cells, and white cells.

These new white cells will be the foundation of a reconfigured cancer-free immune system. Autologous transplants have the best chance for a smooth ride — your body won't reject its own stem cells (a condition called graft versus host disease, or GVHD). The body (host) and the stem cells (graft) recognize each other, and quickly form a partnership to get the body on track again.

The second type, an allogenic transplant, is riskier. The stem cells come from a related donor, usually a sibling. The quality of the match is determined by a protein (HLA) marker. The best outcome happens when all ten markers match, though you can go ahead with as few as six.

The third type is a matched unrelated donor transplant (MUD). For the roughly 70 percent of patients who do not have a donor in their family, this option is their hope for more years of life. However, GVHD is more severe for these patients. All this depends on the quality of the match, and with a good one (8/10 or higher), survival rates are approaching those of related donor transplants.[6]

Radiation is used to shrink cancer and limit complications that can arise from more extensive surgery. Treatments begin with a tattoo — not some bizarre initiation ritual into the club, but a target to line up the radiation beam, so it consistently hits the tumor in every treatment (and there can be upwards of thirty or forty of those treatments). Fortunately, radiation treatment is fast, taking only a few minutes under the machine (though, the larger the area, the longer the time). There is still the travel to and from the hospital, finding parking (always stressful!), waiting your turn, and being delayed if the machine is down for maintenance, so appointments require at least a few hours of your day.

Radiation has advanced dramatically since its inception, when cobalt was used to blast the body into the then slim chance of survival. Now, the beam is narrow and shaped three dimensionally to the tumor. Computers can even adjust for slight movement from breathing — one simply has to lie still on the table, which elevates and slides you into position while the machine rotates around you. Lying still is both easier and harder for head and neck cancer patients. It's easier because a full head mask made of plastic mesh clamps you to the table. It's harder because, for many, this experience triggers claustrophobia. Some patients understandably panic and feel they cannot go through with it. I'm often called in to help in these situations, and am continually impressed with how well patients end up coping.

Radiation accumulates, it builds up in the area of the body treated and continues to work for weeks after the final session is done. This is why a follow-up scan, to determine if the radiation shrank the cancer, is not scheduled until at least six weeks after the last session.

Side effects from radiation and chemotherapy can include skin changes (such as itching, peeling, and blistering), diarrhea, fatigue, hair loss, nausea, repressed sexual desire, neuropathy (nerve damage), and impaired digestion. This all depends on what area of the body receives radiation, and what type of chemo is used. Both chemo and radiation can result in infertility, so if you would like to have children, sperm and egg banking are worth considering before treatment begins.

Targeted therapy is among the most advanced treatments. Instead of hitting all rapidly growing cells like chemo does, it targets specific molecules involved in cancer growth. This may require changing the body's hormonal balance, which can be very effective but has its dark side; weight gain, change in moods and energy, inability to sleep, racing thoughts and a host of physical issues. Some joke that the burst in energy and mental clarity is worth it. They rearrange their closets and accomplish tasks that would take weeks, on little or no sleep. However, this manic behavior can be hard on marriages and families. Why, with this list, would you consider targeted or hormone therapy? Because it can drastically and quickly shrink tumors, giving cancer a powerful punch to bring it down to size for chemotherapy to mop up. Support is also available to help you cope with these side effects, helping couples stay connected and ride the emotional waves of a treatment that compromises communication, intimacy and, in some cases, a person's sanity.

Biological therapy works to enhance your immune system. These are sophisticated and targeted drugs, which include Rituxan for non-Hodgkin's lymphoma and Herceptin for breast cancer. Other drugs increase the white blood cell count or stimulate the production of platelets, which enables blood to clot properly. While on the cutting edge, more and more of these biological drugs are emerging as standard treatment options in centers around the world.

❧

WHEN HOPE FADES

WHAT IF TREATMENT DOESN'T WORK? ARE THERE OPTIONS? A STRONGER chemo may be available, but its effectiveness could be compromised because of the poor condition of the patient, and because cancer can become resistant to treatment. It is in this situation that patients sometimes consider extremely dangerous procedures, hoping they will be among the few who survive. Some will travel the world to receive alternative therapy, determined to extend their lives until the next breakthrough. These breakthroughs are coming — staggering advances have been made in understanding the genome,[7] using light to modify cells,[8] and employing nanotechnology to treat cancer.[9,10] However, the reality is that while overall survival rates have doubled in the last forty years (meaning life has been extended significantly), at a population level, things are going to get a lot worse. As more countries catch up in industrial development, they will also find their cancer levels increase.[11] Despite the billions of dollars poured into research, cures have not improved for most cancers and prevention remains a challenge.

When the straits are truly dire, when death is imminent, many still reach for that slim hope of a trial drug or extremely aggressive chemo. They do this without realizing how much suffering these paths entail. Cancer can make patients understandably desperate for their days to continue and for normality to return, but this can also result in living under the tyranny of hope — a hope that sabotages the opportunity to use death for the most profound shift possible — affirming the power of love, releasing this life with gratitude, and embracing the next with anticipation. That sounds like an impossible task. How can we let go of those we love? How can we anticipate what feels like oblivion? The answers to these most difficult questions have been lived out again and again by the remarkable people I have the privilege to support.

CHAPTER 3

WITNESSING IMMORTALITY

Surely God would not have created such a being as man, with an ability to grasp the infinite, to exist only for a day! No, no, man was made for immortality.

— ABRAHAM LINCOLN

JOSH

AT FOURTEEN, JOSH WAS THE YOUNGEST PATIENT WE'D SEEN, ONE OF our favorites, and not just because of his youth. Josh's spirit was contagious, his optimism a treasure, his graciousness ... his graciousness humbled us all. Never did he complain. In fact, he made a point to try to brighten everyone's day. He'd invite me to play Little Big World, a video game in which a small character made of sackcloth and yarn becomes a hero, facing insurmountable foes in a hand-stitched world that looks like a scrapbooker's dream. Little Big World — it suited him perfectly, with his diminutive stature, shrunken all the more by towering IV poles, laden with pumps and tubes. Because of his irrepressible kindness, Josh was the hardest to care for. Nurses, heartbroken by his grace and cheer, would quietly cry in the chart room. Doctors would pause in the hallway to collect themselves. We all knew his chances were slim.

Josh was having a MUD, a matched unrelated donor transplant. An only child, he had no compatible donor in his family. And his match wasn't perfect: 8/10 variables — good odds, but still risky. We've seen others survive; we've bought them a few years. That's the hope, buying time until new breakthroughs come. Josh had no choice. Not to try meant death within a month. He was willing to face the perils, and seemed inspired by the spunk of the animated character on the screen.

"Besides," he said nonchalantly, "if I die, maybe I'll get another life."

Into the danger he went — weight loss, diarrhea, vomiting, chemo, chemo, and more chemo, all to eradicate his immune system so we could, at 3:00 a.m., infuse him with a new one. The procedure looks so much less grand than the name. It hardly feels like a transplant. The stem cells are warmed in a portable sink, which gently rocks them to distribute the heat. The cells are then infused through the IV. The room is crowded — two doctors, a transplant technician, the nurse, and his parents — all silent as they watch for signs of reaction: rigors, fever, redness in the skin. And there lies Josh, small in the bed, smiling at his mother who rocks and silently prays.

"Don't worry, Mom, I'm a fighter."

It goes smoothly. No reaction, no bumps. Sighs of relief. It took barely twenty minutes. And now, the magic. Stem cells course through his body communicating with every vessel and organ, seeking out the area most in need of repair. There they set up camp, analyze the situation, and begin production of whatever the body requires at that moment — in this case, an entire immune system. New white blood cells will defend Josh against the myriad microbial enemies that swarm not only the outward environment of our world, but the inner environment of our bodies. Health is a constant balancing act, and now the enemy within is the most dangerous. Bacteria, which normally exist in symbiotic truce with our biology, soon take the advantage. With no immune system to protect him, they grow out of control. Josh's body is transformed into a war zone, while microscopically, a few newborn white blood cells take on the swarm. Little Big World — he is it.

Josh is fine for the first few days. We don't expect to see the struggle until about day fourteen, by which time the body realizes it has a foreign invader — a new immune system, but not of its own creating. The battle ensues between an infused ally and the flesh that does not recognize it. Graft versus host disease starts with a fever, then skin irritation. The liver is compromised; the gut takes a beating. Pneumonia, mucositis … the list goes on and on. Steroids are administered to combat these trials, and ironically, immunosuppressant drugs are brought in to tame the very stem cells we have infused. While this battle rages in Josh, he plays his game: a valiant and fragile rag doll character, going against dragons and robots and alligator-infested pits. It was the best therapy he could have.

One day the nurse called. "David, Josh is having a hard time with GVHD. His skin is itchy and flaking off, he can't get much sleep. Can you try Therapeutic Touch? It might help."

Therapeutic Touch is essentially a non-contact energy treatment. Developed by nurses, it is based on the understanding that we not only have a biological anatomy but also an energetic one. The results are wonderful: accelerated healing, deep relaxation, and a subtle rebalancing that can boost the body's natural wisdom. The name is a bit of a misnomer; I rarely touch the patient, instead moving my hands three to six inches above the body. While staff thought it controversial at first, over the years we've found it very effective in relieving the adverse effects of chemotherapy. We'll explore that in chapter 12.

His mom was sitting by the bed, nervously rocking. Josh was not quite as chipper as usual.

"I hear you're going through one of those bumps we talked about," I said. Bumps. What an understatement! Josh looked like he was molting — GVHD had ravaged his skin, which now flaked from him, head to toe.

I explained the procedure, and Josh agreed. Therapeutic Touch turned out to be very effective. It was one of the few things that could relax him and relieve the itching. But the infections were now overwhelming his diminutive form. Kidney failure turned his eyes the color of his sackcloth avatar. Limbs bloated with excess fluid. He became less and less animated. I treated Josh daily, watching him deteriorate, until one day I came in and the bed was empty.

The nurse's eyes were moist, her voice trembling. "He's in ICU. They were wondering if you could go down … things don't look good."

The curtain was closed. Another nurse sat pensively at the desk. She stiffly smiled as I approached. This case was clearly difficult for her, too. We normally would send him to the children's hospital next door, but Josh required a different level of care. And that care had run out. He was now on life support. The new stem cells, full of promise and potential, had been destroyed by the cancer; liver, kidneys, lungs, heart, bowels — they were all failing.

I pulled the curtain. Josh, so small in the bed, was dwarfed even more by the wall of monitors above him. His family gathered in grief: uncles, aunts, grandparents, cousins, mom, and dad. I stood alone on the other side of his bed, looking into their sorrowful eyes.

"Thanks for coming, David. We were wondering if you could give him one more treatment. It was the only thing that seemed to relax him."

"Of course. Of course." So many times I've given Therapeutic Touch to those in pain, with nausea, in distress. In this situation, at death, it is especially humbling. I am entering a soul's essence, the vital energy of a consciousness about to transition to the next world. When I close my eyes to center myself, there is a shift in the room. The family seems to recede as I move my hands above his frail body. Opening through the heart's presence, I listen and find fear. So alone, so overwhelmed. We're all here, Josh. I infuse my thoughts with compassion. We're all with you, your whole family. Feel their love. Feel God's love. We're all with you. And send the love in. As the tears well up, send the love in, and don't shrink back when it becomes hard. Hold the grief, hold the fear, and honor the humanity of it all. Honor the love.

I look up. Across the bed from me is a face I know and would never have expected to see — my best friend, who is also the family's pastor. He is looking into my eyes with great love and compassion as I quietly weep.

"It's all right, David. Keep going," he says.

With that affirmation, I close my eyes again and move into Josh's field. The fear is gone. A peace and depth fill the room, and I am able to send

Josh the message he knew already. God will receive you, the love and the angels will receive you, and you will be more safe and alive than you ever were here. We'll always be with you, Josh. Your family's love is always part of you. It's safe to go.

The treatment over, I look up again. The room has shifted back to its normal proportions. My friend is smiling through his tears. The family waits in silence.

"I felt fear at first, but now I believe he knows you are here, that he is loved." There could be no greater message for them.

After embracing, Josh's parents asked if they could have a few minutes alone with him while the machines are shut off. We quietly left the room. It didn't take long.

They emerged trembling, aware, exhausted, and so, so sad. We all knew Josh was free, not only of suffering but also of the limitations of life on this level. And we sensed he was so much more as well. Just as the fragile character in Josh's game overcame incredible odds through the guidance of the player's unseen hand, we knew God had guided Josh's course and shaped his character. He was now shining, enhanced and embraced by nothing less than the Divine Love of the universe. Because Josh was — is — an emanation of that love, he continues in the journey of evolutionary consciousness, encountering new challenges and adventures in a spiritual body, so unlike ours. He now understands how God had been within his humble human form all along. He is now one among the billions who travel this mystery, this little big world, becoming the hero of his journey and the hero of our hearts. We would walk with that assurance out of the valley of the shadow of death, but not out of the shadow of grief. That wisdom, that pain was for us to hold for quite a while, learning to allow it to shape us, to deepen our humanity, to help us live with renewed awareness of the gift of life.

We embraced. We gathered once again around his bed. We prayed, giving thanks for this young light. The family spent time with his body, the shell of what was. And I returned to my office to weep, before moving on to the next patient.

IMMORTALITY THROUGH LOVE

JOSH, HIS PARENTS, THE STAFF ... WE WERE ALL CHANGED. ALL OF US evolved through this tragedy. What do I mean by this? Josh's cancer cracked us open to love more deeply, to be compassionate witnesses in his journey. In doing so, we resonated more accurately with the consciousness of God, in whom we are eternally connected, through whom love becomes something even death cannot break. While we felt helpless and heartbroken, we were standing on holy ground. It is our privilege to know such love. It is also our destiny to become it.

Love is more than an emotion. It is divine essence, for God is love. This is the very process and product of our conscious evolution — the expansion of our souls to greater levels of being. Think about this for a moment. Love causes us to resonate with the Divine, shifting the frequency of our consciousness to be more in tune with the underlying spiritual reality of who we truly are — not this limited mortal flesh, but an immortal, glorious light. Can you imagine evolving into that kind of entity? Even harder, can you accept that death is ultimately required for this evolutionary step to take place? If only it didn't have to happen through such ordeals as cancer. If only suffering and loss could be removed from the equation. It is here that spirituality has such a vital role to play. It is here that we learn to love our suffering self with a tenderness from which deep meaning will be born. It is here that faith in a loving God, and confidence that you are, indeed, wired for immortality, makes it possible to do more than endure suffering — it makes it possible to shine even brighter through it.

We are all immortal. That can seem like a distant hope, an abstract promise when you lose someone you love. All you know is the pain you feel here, now. Even when the comfort of the afterlife brings you the assurance that you will see your loved ones again, that day entails your dying as well. What a gift, then, when the light of heaven peeks through in our darkest hour, allowing us to witness this transformation from mortality to immortality. There is no greater privilege than accompanying the dying, to witness a soul's transition from this world to the next. There is no greater heartbreak either. The capacity to hold these two extremes in the cradle of compassion is what determines the quality of our presence. It is what determines the depth of care we embody, and ultimately it becomes our practice, our rehearsal for that day when each of us dies. We fall asleep to this world and awaken to that which is beyond the poverty of words.

My role is to incarnate that compassionate presence, and to do so with sensitivity and awareness of the tapestry of faith. This is not a quality that emerges from training, ego, or intellect. We experience it through our own suffering and redemption, which means you have to know brokenness to be a conduit of grace.

Chaplains are there to support such spiritual vitality, that quality of engagement in suffering that deepens and honors everyone's humanity, staff and patients alike. We help to make hospitals places of human care, even though they are centered in disease care. Fifteen years working on a cancer unit has provided me with many opportunities for this to develop.

My studies in world religions and philosophy, being taught by Anglican, Lutheran, Catholic, Baptist, and United Church clergy, Taoist priests, Buddhist monks, rabbis and a good number of atheist professors, has helped cultivate the skill to support people of all faiths and those who have none. To some, I am a welcome guest. Their faith is foundational in getting them through the illness, and I bring the church's comfort through the practice of prayer and sacrament. Approximately a third of patients I see are Roman Catholic, so an essential aspect of spiritual assessment is determining if they would like to receive Holy Communion and the Anointing of the Sick. This is important as Catholic culture often sees the anointing as "last rites," despite the church's efforts to reframe it according to its proper historical roots — as a ritual to strengthen faith and hope throughout the illness trajectory.

For others, though, the presence of the chaplain can trigger guilt, ambivalence, or hostility. The church represents a repressive and harmful structure in their lives. Acknowledging that pain without any defense is critical to creating a space wherein these people can tell a member of the clergy how deeply offended and outraged they are. Even though I am a Lutheran pastor, I represent "church" in all its expressions. Sometimes the best thing I can do is be a sponge for their anger. Pain cannot heal until it has a voice.

And what pain that is. Scandals and corruption, exploitation and bloodshed; the church is as human an institution as any. All the more obscene, though, as it does so in the name of God, a name used through the centuries as a judicial threat meting out reward and punishment. Such an image is impotent to heal our wounds, and heretical to whom Jesus is. Against this is a deeper wisdom within Christianity, one that understands God is love, independent of copyright. While God comes to us in a profoundly personal and compassionate way, that theistic manifestation is a layer upon the transcendent nature of the Divine, far beyond human comprehension. As such, I like theologian Paul Tillich's preference to refer to God as the "Ground of Being," an idea Karen Armstrong draws on as well in her efforts to heal our image of the Divine:

> A God who kept tinkering with the universe was absurd; a God who interfered with human freedom and creativity was a tyrant. If God is seen as a self in a world of his own, an ego that relates to a thought, a cause separate from its effect, he becomes a being, not Being itself. An omnipotent, all knowing tyrant is not so different from earthly dictators who make everything and everybody mere cogs in the machine which they controlled. An atheism that rejects such a God is amply justified.[12]

All this becomes the backdrop to what appears to be simple, pleasant introductions between chaplain and patient. The question becomes how to engage another in crisis while aware of these cultural undertows. Humor can help. "They call me the high priest around here," I say, towering six foot eight above their bed, "but really my role is to simply help you in the experience of your illness." I may pull up a chair, ask how they're holding up, if we're treating them well; gently building the relationship, winding gradually through the labyrinth of their inner world.

Whatever their affiliation and theology or lack thereof, the key is allowing patients and families to lead, honoring their struggle, questions, and conclusions. As they experience this respect, they allow our alliance to grow and take shape. This is for everyone. Chaplains are mandated to respect and support all people in their own faith, whether the person is a Christian, Jew, Moslem, atheist … or a witch.

A Vision in the ICU

A YOUNG WIFE WAS IN DESPAIR AS MACHINES BREATHED FOR HER HUS-band in the intensive care unit. It was midnight when I arrived and introduced myself to her. Her response was awkward but honest: "I don't think you'll be able to help us. We're Wiccan."

I had noticed her pendant, a five-pointed star representing earth, air, fire, water, and spirit. Recognizing this helped start a conversation about the connection between spirituality and hope, while demonstrating respect for her faith. We discussed the situation, the story stumbling from her heart of how this wonderful young man succumbed to a severe infection, how hope unraveled with each unsuccessful antibiotic, and then cancer was discovered. Too late … all too late.

She broke with grief, and then produced a small pouch from her pocket containing seven stones, each of a different material and color. "I wanted to perform the prayers," she said through her tears, "but now I don't know what to do." These prayers involve placing a stone over each chakra, the energetic centers of consciousness. Collectively they form the interface between the body and spirit, between biography and biology. Through the prayers a signature of each chakra is written upon the stones — the life of the person resonates in them.

"I would be honored to do that with you, if you like."

"Really?" She was confused and touched that a Christian minister would be aware of, let alone encourage a pagan rite.

"Sure. Let's go in, I'll tell the nurse what we're doing and pull the curtain for privacy. This is important."

The columns of instruments rose about him like a technological forest, lines and hoses and tubes rooting him to the temporary tree of life. The dim light of the room filtered through the drawn curtain, while the light from LED displays cast a cool, moon-like glow upon his face. Taking a moment by his side, we simply breathed, the chirping of the monitor fading to the background of awareness. The stones were placed; the prayers were said, giving thanks for his body which had served him in this journey. Therapeutic Touch also assisted in the ritual, which was similar to her own understanding of energy fields and consciousness. Smoothing and grounding the flow of his biofield, the key here was to compassionately connect and impart full presence. Body and spirit are wise in the ways of dying; I did not have to direct his in any way. In fact, as always, the recipient leads the treatment, not the practitioner, all the more at the edge of life.

Soon afterwards, their fourteen-year-old son and the patient's mother arrived. I offered support for them, and together we stood at the bed as life support was removed. Their son demonstrated keen awareness of their beliefs, and embraced his mother as his father breathed his last. Then, coming to the opposite side of his bed, he kissed his father's forehead and thanked him for his love. Silence and admiration filled his mother's eyes as she gazed through tears at this young man. And then, his eyes filled and a smile broke out as he looked back at his mother.

"I can see him! He's right beside you!" Their son's face shone with the vision, and his mother's with astonishment. They embraced as I stood by, witnessing love.

CHAPTER 4

FORGING MEANING

Adversity introduces a man to himself.

— ALBERT EINSTEIN

WHY ME?

WHEN PATIENTS ARE DIAGNOSED WITH CANCER IN THEIR EIGHT-ies, we tend to feel they at least had a long life. In their seventies, it feels like there should be more living to do, and we may still be able to extend their years through treatment. As patients get younger, it gets more difficult. A diagnosis of cancer just after retirement feels like a cruel joke. Received in their fifties, and it robs them of seeing their grandkids. In their forties, a vibrant life is cut short. In the thirties, a young family loses a parent. The twenties, and cancer steals a life before it's time. Any younger crushes us beyond words.

There is no good age, and each diagnosis brings the question to the lips of parents who will outlive their child and to people who never imagine cancer can happen to them: Why me? What could I have done? Did I miss vital signs along the way? It is the proverbial question of humanity in the face of suffering. We ask it when diagnosed and throughout the illness trajectory. It is the search for meaning, a groping in the dark for something to make sense of life turned upside down.

Why me? The question is a sign of spiritual distress. Life is suddenly fragile; everything held dear is in jeopardy. Spiritual distress may be defined as a disturbance in a person's belief system, a disruption in the life principle pervading a person's entire being, which integrates and transcends one's biological and psychological nature.[13] We've passed the boundary of our comfort zone. Ahead lie chaos and a new creation (the two always go hand in hand). Spiritual distress is expressed through the big questions: Is God punishing me? Does my life have meaning? Did I do something to cause this? What will happen to me when I die? What if I don't measure up?

People tend to answer these questions in two ways: either it is part of God's plan, or it is not. If it is your destiny, it can leave you feeling both terrified and comforted, for destiny is an expression of both dread (will I ever be able to avoid suffering if it is my fate?) and hope (God must have a purpose in this nightmare). Here's where our image of God will be reflected by the limits of our language. Destiny reflects a severe God who, through some wisdom beyond our ability to comprehend, can use cancer for our betterment. After all, isn't imagining a God in control despite the world's suffering (or even through it) better than meaningless sorrow? If the image of God is not sufficient to hold the experience, it can result in leaving religion behind. As one parent put it, "If my faith demands I accept a 'loving' God who causes such suffering in my child, then I'll have nothing to do with it."

If God does not cause the suffering, but simply allows it, then that implies God's tacit approval of the condition. Again, an intolerable impasse is reached. The resulting anger can reduce faith to ashes, which smolder for a lifetime.

Perhaps it is karma, the cause-and-effect rule of the universe that balances the scales, even if over several lifetimes. If so, are we resigned to suffer the effects of actions we are not even aware of? If the moral law of the universe is "what goes around comes around," then must we resign ourselves to this consequence? This perspective can both empower and exhaust the human spirit: empower because of the belief that through suffering our souls are somehow being refined, and exhaust because understanding karma in this way leaves us feeling destined to repeat the cycle of suffering.

Of course, one doesn't have to wrestle with such existential questions. Many are more pragmatic: Did I get cancer because of the choices I made in life? Have I orchestrated my own downfall? Did I get cancer because I worked with toxic chemicals? Was it caused by my negative thoughts and feelings? What is the emotional influence on this outcome? How can I change so I don't feed it with my own psychodynamic and energetic poison? Does biography become biology? Is it my fault? These questions are statements of responsibility and helplessness, for how can we ever understand the web of life we have spun? And, in a larger context, how can we ever protect ourselves from the hidden variables of genetics, environment, chaos, and coincidence?

Or, maybe it just is. This statement can be profoundly wise and absurdly simple. Why me? Why not. For people in this camp, spending energy wrestling with God is a waste of energy. Perhaps it's best simply to resign ourselves to the situation, get down to business, and leave the ultimate questions to the philosophers.

This question, "Why me," is essential to ask but impossible to answer. It is part of the required wrestling with mortality and must not be satisfied by anyone who has the privilege of supporting you in your experience of cancer. We are so tempted to offer answers, which often do little more than ease our own anxiety. I call them spiritual clichés, and I'm as guilty as the next person for uttering these assurances. They flow from clumsy efforts at empathy: "Everything has a reason." "God has a purpose in this." "You won't be given more than you can handle." Really? Does God believe in us so much more than we believe in ourselves that He would bestow on us this cross? We should be cautious with such an ordination.

A REALITY CHECK

WHY DO WE GET CANCER? NO SHORTAGE OF AUTHORS ON SPIRITUALITY and healing will say it arises from the aberration caused by our disconnection from love. We internalize the message that we are unlovable, then reinforce that message by being unloving. The energetic dissonance in our consciousness then ripples out through the cells, resulting in a tumor (a process I'll explore later in the book). However, before jumping to a spiritual reason for developing cancer, let's first take a more practical approach and look at what's obvious.

Cancer is a disease associated with aging. Almost 90 percent of all cancer diagnoses are in people over the age of 50, and half of those over the age of 70. While the causes are multifactorial and not fully understood, a main one is simply that more people are living longer, but doing so in an environment that has become unhealthy.

We need to own up to the mess we've made: we have created an incredibly toxic world, both physically and psychically. The entire planet is out of balance directly due to our consumption and waste, and cancer is just part of the price we pay. Species are dying off thousands of times faster than the natural extinction rate. Fertility is plummeting due to endocrine-disrupting chemicals like bisphenol A. Autism spectrum disorders soared from 1 in 166 to 1 in 68 in the past fifteen years.[14] To say an individual develops cancer due to lack of love, while they are swimming in such cultural and environmental poison (and doing so through a longer lifespan), not only makes healing through right thoughts simplistic and naive, it is an insult to our impending mortality. It is an abdication of our primary spiritual responsibility to be good stewards of the earth. Everything is connected. We cannot restore balance and healing to the body without also restoring it to each other and the planet. And time is running out.

Cancer rates have risen exponentially since the Industrial Revolution, and may increase another 50 percent by 2020.[15] We are also seeing cancers common in older populations now afflicting young adults and children. Globally, cancer is second only to cardiovascular disease, striking one in three.[16] While the Industrial Revolution accelerated the spread of this disease, it was World War Two that turned it into a plague. Since 1945 over eighty thousand unregulated chemicals have been released into the environment.[17] Even those that are not cancerous have been found to become so as they interact with other elements, a process we are only beginning to understand. Add to this global desertification, pollution of groundwater, accelerated extinction of species, human population growth.... It becomes clear that we are quickly tipping the balance of sustainable life.

Yet, we are not powerless. We do participate in the unfolding of our health; with every choice we take a step toward supporting the body or compromising it. It is vital to remember that 50 percent of cancers are preventable.[18] Even more startling, a 2008 *Pharmaceutical Research* document states, "Only 5–10% of all cancer cases can be attributed to genetic defects, whereas the remaining 90–95% have their roots in the environment and lifestyle. The lifestyle factors include cigarette smoking, poor diet (fried foods, red meat), alcohol consumption, UV exposure (which includes tanning beds as well as sun exposure), environmental pollutants, toxins in products, obesity, and physical inactivity."[19,20]

In a toxic world, it's good to know there are many things you can do to prevent cancer, or at least fortify yourself should the diagnosis befall you. Still, the sting is acute, especially when you've led a healthy lifestyle and done everything right. You get hit with lung cancer, though you never smoked,[21] or a brain tumor, though you don't own a cell phone.[22] We do know some things about how thoughts, emotion, and stress compromise the immune system and contribute to creating a biological environment conducive to disease. This understanding has resulted in a field of research called psychoneuroimmunology, which explores how chronic negative emotions can contribute to an increase in disease and speed death, while positive emotions support disease tolerance and increase the likelihood of health returning.[23] Before diving into the mind-body connection, though, we need to address health on the most practical level: diet, exercise, and sleep. These fundamental factors form the tripod of health, and have a massive influence upon our body. Managing them well will also have a great effect on improving overall well-being. As simplistic as it may seem, when it comes to resistance to disease and resilience if it hits, movement, rest, and healthy food are the best place to start.

You can't be completely safe, though. Given the toxic environment we've created, both within ourselves and around us, there exists within every person the potential for cancer to develop. In fact, most adults are walking around with cancerous cells right now, but these are held in check by the immune system, so they never grow out of control. As the body ages, metabolic resilience also breaks down, resulting in a vulnerability to cancer's growth and an inability to keep those tiny tumors in check.

In addition to this are the significant social determinants of health. Cancer rates among the poor have consistently been higher than average, and over half of cancer deaths occur in less developed countries. This is even worse for women. Worldwide, cervical cancer accounts for 13 percent of female cancers, yet 85 percent of these cases occur in developing countries. The contributing factors escalate layer upon layer — concentration of population, lack of sanitation, stigma, lack of access to preventative health services and contaminated living environments chief among them.[24]

The conclusion is clear: While there are natural genetic mutations or errors in cell division that give rise to the occasional tumor, while thoughts do affect our immune system and resilience to disease, cancer arises from a complex network of factors, chief among which are a longer lifespan and an increasingly unhealthy environment. This ought to reframe all initiatives to eradicate the disease. While billions of dollars are poured into research, we fail to admit to the public, and to ourselves, that there can be no cure until we change our entire civilization. Research is vital and will provide options; amazing breakthroughs will come in our lifetime, but these are part of a larger shift in civilization that will radically alter our species.[25] The individual choices we all have at our disposal — addressing poverty, eating and living well, and reducing environmental toxins, will be far more effective and affordable. We should not wait until a diagnosis before choosing them.

All this is not to diminish the power of love and forgiveness in affecting the body, but when it comes to terminal cancer, most of the patients I've seen who healed their hearts, restored their connection to love, and released the pain they had carried for decades, still died of the disease. But they died more whole and complete, so in that sense they died healed, though not cured — such a better thing, to leave this world heart whole than to hang around years longer never knowing that freedom.

Even with the growing knowledge of how improved standards of living, lifestyle, diet, physical activity, and avoiding tobacco can dramatically improve one's resilience to cancer (and improve odds of successful treatment), patients often fall back on the concept of an external, all-powerful God who both ordains cancer as a fire through which we will draw closer to Him, and the rescuer who will provide the cure. Such a manipulative divine strategy speaks of our fear and search for meaning, not of the loving God of the universe. Studies on religiosity and coping have actually found a negative correlation between the two.[26] I've also experienced this: often, the more strict and doctrinal a person's faith, the higher the risk of maladaptive religious coping — more fervent prayer, more struggle to discern God's will, and then to do the right thing and receive God's favor. Those with a strong faith conviction may still question where God is when suffering, and may see their illness as punishment for life choices. This can result in feeling anger toward God for being so forsaken. This notion, that God gives us trials as a form of discipline, is called a theology of divine retribution. It assumes that God blesses those who are faithful and punishes those who sin. So, the bargaining begins — prayers and petitions for this one life to be spared. Wouldn't it be wonderful if it worked so simply? Maybe it's better that it does not.

George

AT AGE SIXTY-SEVEN GEORGE HAD JUST RETIRED FROM HIS SUCCESSFUL business. He had a wonderful family, a beautiful home, he traveled the world with his loving wife, and was a man of faith who enjoyed his church community. But now that faith terrified him, because he had just received exactly what he had prayed for.

Six months earlier his five-year-old granddaughter was diagnosed with astrocytoma, an aggressive brain tumor. Prayer chains and church vigils had been held, well wishes and casseroles poured in to the home. And, in the quiet of a grandfather's heart, a secret prayer was lifted up with more conviction and intensity than he had ever known: If it is at all possible, dear God, let me take the cancer from her. Give it to me. I've lived a good life and I love her so much. George sat in the counseling room with me sobbing, shaking, as he confessed for the first time this terrifying request and its consequence.

His granddaughter's cancer had been successfully treated with surgery and radiation. They had just received news the week before that her recovery had been admirable, and her discharge was imminent. Hope restored, the family celebrated the gift of her life and the joy of sharing it with her — all except her grandfather. He had just been diagnosed with astrocytoma, but for him, it was inoperable.

"I'm so scared. I'm so scared. What have I done?! How can I speak of this to my wife, my kids? I can't ever let them know. They're going to watch me die, they're going to stand at my grave. It's my fault." The pain of that was more than George could bear. He folded upon himself, limp and crumpled in the chair. Tear-swollen eyes pleaded to heaven. "What if I hadn't prayed? Would my granddaughter be dying now instead? Is this what God has planned?"

He wanted an answer — he wanted it verified by a man of God that heaven had, indeed granted his prayer for the sake of his granddaughter. And, unspoken, was the question: could he escape this fate for the sake of the suffering his family would endure. Was there a way out?

"George, this is a terrifying situation for you, and it can even leave you scared of the power of your own thoughts. You're left feeling trapped, having to accept God's answer to your prayer, wanting to escape it, and then feeling guilty for even thinking that because you fear the cancer might go back to your granddaughter. Is that what this feels like?"

He nodded slowly. "Exactly, I'm trapped. And I can't take it back now. What do I do?"

I asked the same of myself. What can be said to a person in this situation? Did I even believe his prayer had that power, that God would do such a thing? It really didn't matter, though. The only thing that did matter was what George believed.

"I have no idea what God's plan is for you," I responded, after taking a moment to listen between his words, "but if you were able to take your granddaughter's cancer upon yourself, it speaks of the astonishingly powerful love you have for her. Your longing to escape this fate does not diminish that love in any way, for it also comes from the desire to protect her, not only from physical suffering, but from the emotional pain of watching you die. On top of this is imagining her ever finding out you had this prayer answered — the responsibility she would feel for getting sick and having you pay the price."

George was nodding in recognition of how deep the love and subsequent displaced responsibility went.

"So you want to protect her, and your whole family, from that, too. This also comes from your love. The pain of imagining the emotional fallout from this is greater than anything."

Now he was listening, recognizing the ripple effect of a prayer that could be a curse and a blessing.

"George, if you are powerful enough to manifest a prayer like that, then you are also powerful enough to love courageously throughout your dying. You're doing that by sharing this struggle with me. You're finally telling someone. But I want you to consider other factors that may have contributed to this cancer beyond that prayer. There may be more at play here. While astrocytoma can have a hereditary link, that's only in about 5 percent of cases. Its cause, as with most cancers, is unknown, but there are strong correlations with environmental toxins."

"Well, I was in the flooring business," he said. "The off-gassing was really strong, but we didn't know anything about health risks. It just smelled bad. You think that was the cause?"

"I don't know. We may never know. But this would be a good thing to talk about with your doctor. As powerful as your prayer may have been, the environmental factors could be even stronger."

George left still believing that he had brought cancer on himself. But at least he was now willing to tell his family and let them in on his anguish, so they could love him through it.

Is there a reason for everything? A plan or hand that guides us? That does not have to mean that God sets us up for suffering. If anything, God takes extraordinary measures to not violate our free will. Perhaps, from the perspective of heaven, all moments are known, all variables are clear, and all outcomes are secured. There is no mess we could ever create that can thwart the objective of divine will — to have us evolve into love. Unfortunately, it is through our wounds that this objective is best achieved. The cracks lead us to a deeper interior life. Beneath ego and exteriors, gold is waiting, and our hands will be bloodied by the digging. It is in this way that meaning is not found, but forged. It is tempered and hardened in the fire of suffering and grief, shaped by loss and edged with tears. This work of the heart breaks down walls we didn't even know existed, and allows us to feel the connection to each other through our pain. After all, a sorrow shared is half as heavy. All this deepens our humanity and tunes our consciousness, preparing us for the day of our own transformation.

If there is a reason for all the suffering, it lies hidden deep in the mystery beyond our mortality and can wait there for us. While here, let us not abdicate our collective culpability by consigning the mess to God's plan. That gives suffering undeserved nobility. No, we are the ones ennobled, as we use the challenge for the betterment of the world and of our character. This is what is meant, I believe, by the oft misapplied passage from Romans 8:28.

> And we know that in all things God works for the good of those who love him, who have been called according to His purpose.

"According to his purpose" is a call to social transformation, addressing the collective ills of poverty, greed, addiction, and exploitation. It is no exemption from the pleasantries of life, but a promise that as we engage our suffering with wisdom and compassion, we will grow into the likeness of love itself. Perhaps the real question we need to ask, then, is not, Why did I get cancer, but, What am I going to do with it.

CHAPTER 5

SPIRITUALITY

In order to experience everyday spirituality, we need to remember that
we are spiritual beings spending some time in a human body.
— BARBARA DE ANGELIS

I SCARE PEOPLE. AFTER ALL, IF YOU'RE LYING IN A HOSPITAL BED WITH cancer and a chaplain walks in, what's the first thought that pops into your mind? I'm going to die! He's here to check my ticket and see which way I'm going. Often, a person will awkwardly confess, "I haven't been to church in a very long time." To which I will smile, and reassure them that this is not about religion, or even about belief, though we can go there. I'm dropping in to see how they're doing.

It's a frightening ride, plain and simple. My role is not only to support faith, but to help with coping and connecting to the inner strength and wisdom we all have but feel so distant from in a crisis. After all, the point, at life's end, is not to be good or have it all together, but to be real. My job is to help people become as real as possible through cancer. My job is to help them become love — not just to love, but to evolve their consciousness through crisis, discovering that love is the bottom line and courage is their core.

This is done through authentic engagement, by being with a skilled and caring person who can help you go to the places that scare you, by unearthing that which is hidden or suppressed. In doing so, you discover a deeper life. This material of the psyche is massive and includes, in no small part, the experience of guilt — guilt of being the cause of so much worry in loved ones; guilt of not being strong and self-reliant as time and treatment render you weak, incontinent, dependent; guilt of not being able to provide or contribute to the family as before.

So great is this distress that patients often feel they cannot let their family down, so they take all the treatments, even those that will cause extreme suffering and, sometimes, death. Spending so much energy protecting loved ones from these most difficult conversations leaves everyone disconnected. Emotional intimacy becomes the first casualty, at a time when it is needed most. The problem is, when we are unable to be authentically present with ourselves, we cannot be authentically connected to others. We feel too vulnerable, too overwhelmed, and too terrified.

So, it doesn't help when the chaplain walks in. Now the patient feels even more awkward! I'm grateful for the training that taught me how to work with this perception and become a sacred witness, a guide in this journey to the shadowlands of the heart. The task of the witness is not to provide any answers but to assist the individual toward their authenticity, where they can stand in their pain, adapt to their crisis, and connect more deeply. As you practice this, you realize letting go is easier than hanging on to something that wasn't real. By engaging our mortality in this way, we are really engaging our living. This is the spiritual dimension of cancer.

THE NUMINOUS PRESENCE

BUT WHAT IS SPIRITUALITY? EVERYONE IS SPIRITUAL, FROM THE ATHEIST in the foxhole, to the most pious and devout. (It's not true that there are no atheists in foxholes. I've met some who stuck to their principles to the end.) But few are able to express how they are spiritual. This must be the most ineffable quality of consciousness, and we stumble over words as we try to capture its essence. One simply has to Google the term "spirituality" to realize there is no single answer — it is as diverse as the cultures and communities that make up the mosaic of humanity.

Religion has been defined as "the search for significance that occurs within the context of established institutions that are designed to facilitate spirituality."[27] Researchers define spirituality as "the journey people take to discover and realize their essential selves and higher order aspirations,"[28] or a "search for the sacred," or "an individual's internal orientation toward a transcendent reality that binds all things into a unitive harmony."[29] There is no conclusive definition for the term, which is why I'm quite comfortable throwing my own into the pot, and giving it a stir: Spirituality is the immanent and transcendent sense of the numinous that is privately experienced and corporately expressed in every aspect of our humanity.

That deserves some explanation. I like the term "numinous." It means power or presence. First used by the Lutheran theologian Rudolf Otto in his book *The Idea of the Holy*, it refers to something of "daunting awfulness and majesty," while also being "something uniquely attractive and fascinating."[30] This is a personal experience that wells up from within, a surprising desire to be in communion with this presence, even to be consumed by it. Sound familiar? Have you ever felt ecstasy so intense that it seemed you would burst from your body, or encountered a beauty so amazing you longed to disappear in it? Have you ever stood alone in the darkest night and been returned to your ancestral origin by the grandeur of the Milky Way? If you have, you have sampled something of the numinous.

It is *immanent* and *transcendent*. It is both within you and just beyond your grasp, a realization that you are not alone. It catches your breath, sends the imagination reeling to all its dark recesses. Suddenly, you are small and insignificant. Suddenly, you are frail and vulnerable. And yet, you are held in the moment by this "something" that is so much greater. If you reject the idea of a personal God, then call this Meaning, the Now, the awareness that you gaze out, and within, to a universe looking back upon itself. You are the stuff of stars, and the implications are simply staggering.

I recall feeling this the first time I went to explore night photography.

Driving almost an hour from the city to avoid light pollution, I found myself at Peggy's Cove, a well-known tourist spot renowned for its granite rocks, crashing waves, and the famous lighthouse. I parked down from the village. A well-marked winding path led to a monument: the Swissair Flight 111 memorial. On September 2, 1998, a McDonnell Douglas MD-11 crashed into the Atlantic Ocean, killing all 229 passengers and crew. My vision was to capture the Milky Way behind the memorial stone, which had three notches for 111, the flight number.

Standing in the dark, the ocean tide below, feeling the night around me, I imagined how those passengers must have felt, the overwhelming panic as their worst nightmare unfolded with the plane hitting the ocean at over six hundred miles an hour. Looking at the stars above the waves, a prayer rose up with the lump in my throat. I recalled the families and staff I had counseled at the time of the disaster. I wanted the photograph to convey hope that those souls now shone with the stars, as the ancients believed; that they somehow look down on their loved ones. With that intention, I was suddenly filled with fear and trembling, along with a compelling fascination. I contemplated the moment they were transformed through death. The dark received my salty tears, just as the ocean received their bodies, 229 souls dropped into oblivion, suddenly across the veil into wonder.

It was a profound and private moment of spiritual awareness, yet it affected how I related to the world, to my life, and so was corporately expressed. Every aspect of our humanity reveals our level of spiritual attunement. Some of us shine with light and love; some of us smolder. Most are a mixture. Spirituality must be an individual experience, as we can only encounter the world through the filter of our senses and the blinders of our perceptions. But it is always a corporate expression, manifest in how we treat ourselves, each other, and the world. It may be private, but it can never be hidden.

Religion, on the other hand, is corporate, systematic spirituality; corporate in that it is a shared group experience, systematic in that it is structured upon beliefs, rituals and doctrine. The term "spirituality" is actually a modern Western invention. There was no such distinction between what was sacred and what was earthly for most of history. The Divine has always been among us; all thoughts, words, and actions were understood to have repercussions as they affected the relationship we have with that invisible realm, which underpins all existence.

The term "spirit" means "animating or vital principle in man and animals." It comes from the Hebrew *ru'ach* (רוּחַ), meaning "soul, courage, breath." That last word should catch ours. Breath. In the Hebrew scriptures, God is described as breathing life into the clay form of Adam (which literally means, "dirt man," of the earth). In Genesis, the Spirit of God hovers over the waters of chaos. The way "Spirit" is used there is unique in the scriptures, for it describes a hen fluffing her wings over a nest, which is about to cradle new life. It is always female in gender, it is always creative and expansive. It is the breath, the life, and the character of a person. The Hebrew concept of breath also shows up in the masculine name of God: *Yahweh,* which is written as four letters, יהוה, pronounced "Yod, Hey, Vah, Hey."

American pastor and writer Rob Bell has an excellent exploration of this in a video called *Breathe.* In it, he points out that these letters are actually vowel sounds. Breathing sounds. And he points out that when God breathes into you, you are given life. The essence of God (love) flows into you, it sanctifies you, it releases you, it makes you whole, which is the meaning of the word "salvation." This is not a one-time thing — it is a relationship, an ongoing interconnectivity, the inescapable foundation through which we live and move and have our being. Rob Bell remarks, "When a baby is born, what's the first thing it has to do to survive? Take a breath, or say the name of God? At the end of our journey do we die because we can no longer breathe, or because we can no longer say the name of God?"[31]

This awareness is always before me as I visit the sick and dying. I am there not only to support the patient, but also to honor the presence of the Divine, manifest through the breath, especially the moment the breath ceases. With that final exhalation, I am opened, apprehended, aware with fear, trembling, and fascination. This person is about to be transformed, and it is marked by a sound unique to the soul: the final breath. An amazing moment, not only in its quality but also its energy. When we are open to this, there can be a real sense of a person's spirit filling the room, of something vital leaving the body, which we know to our core is now an empty vessel. That person is no longer there. Something essential has changed, and we fundamentally do not know what it is.

MARTHA

I WILL NEVER FORGET MARTHA, WHO LITERALLY AND MYSTERIOUSLY GAVE me the gift of her final breath. I had known her for years. The mother of a parishioner in my church, I recalled visiting with her when I first arrived. I was a young and green pastor in my first metropolitan church, and she was a gracious host, who served excellent pie. It felt a privilege to sit at her bedside with her daughters and their husbands so many years after that pleasant afternoon.

"How long?" her daughters asked. It's an important question. We're looking for signs along the road, some indication of how the journey will unfold, some bearings so we aren't so scared when death arrives.

"Well," I said, "let me give you a lay of the land, so to speak, so you can recognize what's happening and be less anxious. If your mom follows the pattern that most often occurs, we'll notice a few things. Her hands and feet will get very warm and then very cold as the blood moves to the core of her body. As a result, her skin will change color, especially on her fingertips. It's subtle. Her breathing will shift, periods of apnea, or pauses between breaths, getting longer and longer as death gets near. Five seconds, ten, fifteen, even up to thirty or forty-five. This may go up and down, but generally the intervals increase over the hours. When it reaches about thirty seconds you know death could happen any moment.

"Dying is a process, and throughout it she is experiencing shifts in consciousness to deeper and deeper levels of detachment from the body and changes in awareness. Her senses, how her consciousness is mediated through her body, are shutting down, but her sense of hearing may become more acute. She may be listening, even when you whisper. So it's important to sit at her side and tell her you love her. Talk to her so she knows she's not alone. That's actually going to help her feel safe. The medicine helps her feel comfortable, but your love is what makes her feel safe. Then, at the end, she may have a brief surge of awareness, open her eyes and see something we may not. If she does, just tell her you love her and that she can go. Then she will close her eyes, there may be a long pause, and she'll take a final breath, and give up her spirit."

Her daughters listened with rapt attention. This was what they needed to know, this was their orientation to love, aligning their hearts back to full and compassionate presence. It had the opposite effect upon their husbands, who were now looking around nervously, shifting their weight from side to side.

"So, this could take a while, right?" one asked.

"It could be hours, or minutes," I replied. I checked her hands and feet. "She's still warm, her breathing is regular. A little while."

Passing the time with stories is always best. We talked about her life, her strictness with her family, the ways her daughters pushed back, the inevitable dramas, and the deepening of love that sometimes can only grow through strain and difficulty.

Martha's breathing shifted. Five seconds. Ten. Over the hour, we could see the change. So I made an invitation.

"Why don't we gather around her bed now, say the prayers and send her our love?" Hands joined. We all took a deep breath, a moment of silence. "Gracious God, the time is so close. Martha is about to leave us, she's soon going to wake in your presence, to wake in awareness and light and love like she's never known, but has always known her. Enfold her, we pray, in the embrace of an angel. Fill her mind with peace, her heart with love, her body with grace. May she be able to release this body with gratitude for carrying her on the journey, with compassion for its limits, and without regret. We commend her to your care, in the hope that we will see each other again. Martha, if you can hear us, know that you are loved. Feel your daughters' love flowing into your heart, know that you will always be connected."

Another moment of silence. Listen for the words and the movement of what should be next. So much goes on within me as I pray in these situations, and so little, too: breath changes, speed of thought slows, heart opens, vulnerability and strength fill my being. I feel the hand holding mine. Open to the Spirit holding us. Hold the moment. Breathe with her. To manifest the prayer, I must disappear. It's a beautiful privilege.

"Loving God, we fumble for words to express our faith and our fear. As ours fall far short, lead us in those words you taught your disciples ..." Our voices resonate in quiet recitation: "Our Father, who art in heaven, hallowed be Thy Name...." Never in church have I prayed those words as I do at the deathbed. They become a whisper, a hush, a pause pregnant with the *mysterium tremendum*, being in the presence of something so much greater. I am under the stars again.

The prayer is over. I place my hand upon her forehead, my thumb making the sign of the cross as the ancient words flow like baptism's water, once again naming her as so much more than Martha, so much more than mortal. "May God bless you and keep you. May God's light shine upon you and be gracious to you. May God look upon you with favor, and give you peace. You are, and always will be, a child of heaven."

The husbands are the first to break the circle. It's a very intense experience, a difficult emotional weight to maintain. "Well, I'm going to step out for a smoke," says one.

"I'll join you," says the other. Their wives do not protest. There's no doubt of the love, but some are able to stay, and others need to catch a breath, even as the patient is losing theirs.

The energy is different in the room. The pause in breathing is now ten seconds. "Is there any way we can know what it's like for Mom?" one daughter asks. "To be sure she's not in any pain?"

"Yes," I reply. "Notice she's not twitching, her hands are at rest, even her eyes are still beneath her lids. I can also check Martha's field using Therapeutic Touch, to see how her energy is."

They were familiar with my practice of this gentle tool from the church — we used to have classes and even incorporated it into the Eucharist. After receiving Communion, people would often remain at the altar for a brief treatment. Even though it made the service longer (always a risk!), many spoke of how nice it was to have a moment of quiet contemplation and connection with the Spirit.

"Yes, please, that's a great idea."

I breathed quietly by Martha's side, centering and grounding while at the same time getting out of my own way. The goal is to truly "listen" to a person's field. Martha was to lead this encounter; I was to fully show up and respond. My hands hovered above her head, and instantly there was a sensation of a flow, but coming out of her crown, not into it. My heart raced with the realization, Is she going? Is this her spirit? Scanning down her body, there was very little sensation. The biofield was close to her skin, flat and weak. The only spike was at the base chakra, a gentle flowing in. She's dying. She's leaving now, I realized. Even though my curiosity wanted to stay at her head — to feel the soul leave the body would be incredible — out of respect I stepped away and turned to her daughters.

"I think she's leaving us now, there's a flow coming out through the crown of her head." I moved to the window while her daughters came and sat at her side. One gently stroked Martha's forehead. "We love you, Mom. We love you." The apnea had now reached over twenty seconds. And then Martha did something that completely surprised me, even though I had described it moments before. She opened her eyes, turned to her daughter, and gazed with a clarity that saw right into her. "We love you, Mom. Time to go," her daughter said through tears and wonder.

Martha turned her head back to gaze at the ceiling, closed her eyes, and stopped breathing. Ten, twenty, thirty seconds. The final inhalation was deep, but it was the exhalation that made my skin tingle. The name of God. The sound of breathing. The final vowel.

I was gently, suddenly filled with a sensation that rippled through my entire being. Laughter and tears mingled in a release of energy that caught me off guard, made my head light, and snapped the daughters' heads around with a wide-eyed expression.

"That's mother's laugh!" one exclaimed, while her sister beamed with joy through teary eyes.

"Mother's laugh! She's free, she's really free!"

Moments later the two husbands returned and realized what happened. "She's gone?! When did it happen?"

"Just now. Just before you came in."

"Really? Are you OK? We shouldn't have left...."

The other husband spoke up with a wry grin. "Now, Steve, you know she didn't really like us anyway." With that, we all burst into laughter. The daughters shared the story of their mother's spirit touching me, while I stood incredulous and grateful, shaking my head at what I had just experienced.

So many times families are anxious about not being present for the final moment. They skip meals, sleep by the patient's bed, and lie awake at night in fear of not being there for the moment they pledged to witness. But they're not in control; the patient is. Even unconscious and unresponsive, the patient is mysteriously partnering with God in the timing of their transformation. Somehow, baffling alignments will occur, and they will hang on to reach that special date, such as an anniversary, birthday, or significant holiday, despite our expert medical opinion on the hours that may remain. This is why I often ask if there is a significant date coming up. A loved one may be traveling to join the family, racing against time to make that connecting flight or driving through the night to get to the hospital. The patient seems able to exert a mysterious ability to hang on until they arrive. Conversely, if the character of the patient seems to be such that they would rather protect their loved ones, they may go so far as to move them out of the room before they die. That seemed to be the case with Martha and her sons-in-law. It was as if she said, As much as I love you boys, this is a time for my daughters and me. You go out and have a smoke.

To us the influence feels like an idle thought. In hindsight, it causes one to pause and wonder if we have any choice at all! Is everything so guided? In my experience, yes, but not so as to violate our free will in any way. Perhaps the dying person's soul, wiser and more connected than we can comprehend, at the moment of death simply understands us better than we do ourselves.

PART 2

Forgiveness and Grief:
The Journey Is Healing

CHAPTER 6

SECOND TUMOR

My scars remind me that I did indeed survive my deepest wounds.

— STEVE GOODIER

SOMETIMES, A MISTAKE CAN SAVE YOUR LIFE. I WAS GRATEFUL FOR the inexperience of the young technician, who hadn't bothered to read my chart note, but simply proceeded with the ultrasound and was surprised when he saw what looked like something pushing on the dome of my bladder. Despite my explaining that the top half was, in fact, gone as a result of surgery ten years prior, he sent a concerned report back to my doctor, convinced something was wrong. It was on her suggestion I was there, an extra measure in my annual cancer check to ensure all was clear.

Examining the report, she also concluded something was pressing against my bladder and ordered a CAT scan along with blood and urine analysis. Then she sent me on my way without any mind to what must have sounded like the typical patient pronouncement: "I'm fine. It's only scar tissue from the last operation. There's nothing there."

What did bother me, though, were the increasing spells of light-headedness and fainting. I chalked that up to nerves; I always had been insecure about my height, an awkward introvert who cracked his head on the door one too many times. My doctor suggested these were anxiety attacks combined with orthostasis, a common experience of blood not carrying enough oxygen to the brain when one stands up too quickly. On me, that blood has a long way to go! I recall this happening in high school during a band tour: momentarily blind, I stepped off the stage and cut my scalp neatly on a nail while ducking under a partition. To this day I feel the scar as I ponder the mystery of consciousness and how many times I've lost it.

Now twenty-seven and a seminary student in Saskatchewan, this was happening frequently and at the most awkward moments, such as while giving a sermon! It made becoming a minister feel like a complete waste of time. How could I preside at worship if I was going to collapse? Time and time again, despite my head saying I could do this, my body would declare "No!" and literally shut off. Blood pressure dropped, my skin became clammy and pale, the room spun, and down I went. This did more than cause embarrassment and self-doubt, it was also painful and dangerous. I have a long way to fall, and the concussion is, literally, stunning.

I knew public speaking was the number one phobia in our culture, surpassing even death, but surely my response was extreme. As a result, I felt confused, angry, and ashamed. Why continue? Why try to do anything that might make me nervous? Was I a coward, unable to experience the exhilaration and satisfaction of rising to a challenge?

These numerous episodes caused my first wife particular strain. We were a young couple and appreciated any extra income, so I took services whenever I could at remote country churches. While the experience was important, the mileage check was a huge bonus. She, however, couldn't stand it when Sundays meant anxiously waiting for me to crash to the floor. One service was hours from home, providing an opportunity to visit friends for the weekend who lived closer to the parish. She chose to stay at their farm and help out while my friend, another David, joined me for the additional hour-long drive to the service. A lot of self-talk and motivation marked that trip. I needed to prove to myself that I was not only competent for the challenge, but also fit for the call. I was determined we would all have a great experience and connect with that mysterious presence and peace within the heart that worship is meant to cultivate. So, David drove while I silently rehearsed my sermon and secretly prayed to stay conscious.

Smiles and sincere hospitality greeted us at the church, a small white spire in a prairie oasis. The sun speckled off a nearby stream under a patch of trembling aspen. My stomach was also doing somersaults, my head already glistening with sweat. *Not now, not this time*, I thought, as I found the bathroom, splashed cold water on my face, and breathed deeply; no turning back. I put on my vestments and entered the small sanctuary.

Stage fright is an opportunity in disguise, energy to be channeled into a talk to create vitality, engagement, and that elusive, essential experience of inspiration. From the moment of my greeting and the opening words of the liturgy, I could feel a change in my body, an energy and ease that are relaxing and engaging at the same time. I was going to be okay. This was all going to be fine. The opening prayer flowed easily off the page, the scripture readings allowed me a moment to sit and breathe deeply. I gazed out at the tiny congregation, twenty-five elderly faces, people tied to the land. Stories written in their wrinkles made me pause. What could a young student say? Could anything new be heard from me? I should be the one listening to them. I soon would be.

We rose for the Gospel. I read it calmly, confidently, and began my sermon. Then the shift began. I have about five seconds warning before I collapse; the sweat and cold suddenly infuse my skin, the room swirls, and everything goes black. Silence and darkness washed me away before I hit the floor. David later told me that the congregation saw me pause, turn pale, slur incomprehensibly and wilt like overcooked pasta. My head slammed against the piano, then bounced off and hit the organ on my way down. I had struck a chord!

I awoke completely disoriented, unable to move or recall who or where I was. Voices around me slowly penetrated the thick fog. I recognized one: my friend, fighting to stay calm as he called my name. I murmured, raised a finger to show him I was still alive, and then threw up. Now I knew, now I remembered; now I cursed myself for yet another monumental embarrassment. Tears welled up with shame, and I muttered, "I'm sorry. I'm sorry." The congregation compassionately surrounded me, frightened and overwhelmed. David cleaned up my mess. "How long?" I ask.

"You've been out about fifteen minutes," he said. "We called the paramedics; they should be here in a while. You need to lie still." I had no problem with that, my body felt like lead, and I once again passed out.

The ambulance arrived. A light was shining in my eyes, a voice behind it asking, "Do you know your name? Do you know where you are?" My answers were accurate, my senses were clear, but my hope was spent. All I wanted to do was go home.

"You're not going home, David." Another paramedic was behind me, bracing a stiff board against my back. "We're taking you to the hospital, you may have a severe concussion." He then asked, "Is there any fluid from his nose?"

I tell David, "They're checking to see if I cracked my skull." Cerebral fluid would drain from my sinuses. Then I breathed in deeply, rolled my eyes and went stiff. They didn't think it was funny, but at least it was a way I could reassure my friend, and through him, my family, that I was OK.

I was strapped to the board, my head secured with foam pads, and loaded into the ambulance. "Tell my wife I'm OK, that I won't do this again." He thought I was talking about passing out, but I was really talking about my career. I would finish my degree, I silently vowed, but then go on to some desk job, any job, that asked nothing of me but to show up. I was done.

Chit-chat on the way was meant to distract and relax me during the bumpy ride down country roads, but I just wanted to sleep, to escape what had become so much more than humiliation. At the hospital, the pleasant doctor was efficient but concerned; the x-ray showed something odd in my neck, a possible fracture.

"I'm fine, it's just a bump. This has happened so many times, I just need a good night's sleep."

Despite my assurances, he shoved an NG tube down my nose, loaded me onto an air ambulance, and sent me back to Saskatoon with a stern warning: If it was a fracture or break, the slightest movement could render me paralyzed or dead. "Take this situation seriously; don't argue, deal with it!" I barely spoke throughout the flight.

It took several hours for family to arrive, time enough to determine my neck was fine, but my ego had taken a bruising. Once home, the hard lesson of humility unfolded with a crumpled piece of paper found in my pocket a few days later. I read it with stunned amazement: "We're so glad you came down to share God's word with us. We pray you're doing well, and will continue to pray for your recovery. God bless you in your ministry, and we sincerely hope you'll come down again when you're feeling better. We'd love to have you back." Attached was a check, covering the service and mileage both ways. They also paid for the air ambulance. Amazing grace. Their generosity taught me so much that day.

I did go back, months later. I had to thank them for their heartfelt compassion, which provided a profound lesson in God's unconditional love, especially when we stumble and fall. They smiled at the allusion. I got through the sermon and service just fine, and promised, from there on, that I would strap myself into the pulpit with bungee cords and wear a crash helmet.

As David and I drove out of the valley following my second visit, I wondered what was going on. Why would I be calm and collected for one service, and not the next? What were these episodes really about? These questions remained on my mind as the summer rolled by and I prepared for internship. For a solid year, fifty-two Sundays, I would have plenty of opportunities to prove myself and get over what I assumed were panic attacks. If anyone was going to be rendered unconscious through my sermons, it would not be me!

SITTING ON A TIME BOMB

WE LEARNED THE SIGNS WELL: FIRST, MY FINGERNAILS TURNED BLUE, THEN the sweating started along with stomach cramps and diarrhea. A few seconds before I blacked out, a calm set in, vision became distorted, then, finally, unconsciousness. Recovering was awful; hypoxia is a sickening experience. Even ten seconds of oxygen starvation and the brain reacts with nausea, dizziness, weakness, disorientation, and memory loss. You collapse, you vomit, you drag your sorry self to a bed, and you sleep. Altitude sickness is a common cause, but I couldn't accept that my height had any part to play in this affliction.

Because the ultrasound technician in Saskatoon had made a mistake, my doctor ordered subsequent tests, which confirmed this was more than nerves. We sat in her office as she went over the result. Urine analysis showed a strange concentration of catecholamines, residual components of adrenaline. They were over twice the normal limit. And, while there was nothing pushing on my bladder, the CT scan did show a mass near my femoral artery where it split and ran down my right leg. The biopsy conducted a week later, performed under CT imaging, confirmed the suspicion: another tumor had developed. This one provided us with a more accurate diagnosis than was available ten years earlier: an active pheochromocytoma. These are the same as paraganglioma, the first tumor I had at seventeen. When found on the adrenal glands, as over 90 percent of them are, they are called "pheos." When they grow elsewhere in the body, they're called paraganglioma. Less than 10 percent are malignant. Mine appeared to be the most extreme exception: extra-adrenal, metastatic, and metabolically very active.

As years passed, the tumors would reappear, and we would learn that they fell into a gray area: malignant in behavior but not in cellular structure. It would lead me to ask again and again as I reviewed the pathology reports, "Is this cancer, or a benign tumor?" My endocrinologist reminded me that just because they looked different from most cancers, that did not diminish the threat. They spread to other areas of the body, and they definitely threatened my life, so they were malignant. However, he reminded me, their danger lies not only in how they spread, but in how they behave.

These tumors act like a Molotov cocktail. The release of adrenaline is the trigger, signaling the tumor to discharge many times the dosage of dopamine, noradrenalin, and other hormones. The result is catastrophic; most people die instantly. Blood pressure skyrockets, blood vessels burst.

It's as if the entire circulatory system is overloaded with super octane fuel. Symptoms of lesser attacks include racing heart, profuse sweating, poor circulation, diarrhea, and stomach cramps. It fit perfectly. It also meant I had taken my life in my hands every time I stepped into the pulpit, every time I even got excited. I was a time bomb!

I also exhibited an interesting variation on the blood pressure spike. Basically, my BP would jump and then, just as suddenly, bottom out. This explained the fainting and may have saved my life. Blood vessels relaxed in overcompensation for the sudden constriction, causing me to pass out. The blue fingernails, which preceded an attack, were from high levels of calcium blocking my capillaries.

Pheos are rare, occurring in two per million people a year.[32] While they induce what appear to be panic attacks, they are present in less than 1 percent of people with hypertension. The tumors grow slowly, taking ten years or more to reach a size that will show up on a scan. Yet even if only a few inches in size, pheochromocytoma can still be potent. Survival rates are difficult to determine, given how rare it is. If the tumor recurred, the chance of making it to five years was 50 percent. When caught early and successfully removed, one can enjoy a normal lifespan, but the surgical procedure is incredibly dangerous, for the tumor will release its payload with the slightest manipulation. When that happens, survival is unlikely.

Because the first tumor was in my bladder, the catecholamine levels were not elevated — all of the metabolites were flushed out in my urine. But now the second one was on a main artery. The tumor's chemicals would spread rapidly throughout my body, along with any seed cells. Who knew where else it could be growing? Pheochromocytoma are not affected by chemotherapy, and are resistant to radiation. Therefore, the only option for me was surgery. A bomb squad, in other words, would have to go in and defuse this thing. Problem was, no one in the province had done it before. My medical team would have to be assembled and educated on what, to them, was an exotic and fascinating case, but to me was Russian roulette.

I was told to go home and relax. Seriously relax. No more sermons, no exercise, no scary movies, no intimacy, nothing that might excite me, startle me, or trigger the tumor in any way. No joy, no surprises, no worry, no fear, no anger, no stress. No life. To feel could be fatal.

A NEW REASON TO LIVE

IN A MEDICAL CRISIS YOU PLACE YOUR LIFE IN THE HANDS OF THE EXPERTS. They are the ones who understand the mysteries of anatomy, the mechanisms of disease, and the methods of physical healing. No wonder doctors have always been revered. In ancient times their secret alchemy was passed on through fraternities and guilds. Their integrity was sealed by the Hippocratic Oath, a pledge to uphold the ethics and principles of the sacred healing arts, sworn before the gods Apollo, Asclepius, Hygeia, and Panacea. For my doctor and his medical team, that pledge, "to prescribe regimens for the good of my patients according to my ability and judgment, and to never do harm,"[33] resulted in a confession: they didn't know how to treat me. No one had removed a pheochromocytoma before. I was a guinea pig.

Rather than undermining my confidence, I appreciated their honesty, and felt at the center of their care. While I did ask if there were hospitals where they specialized in such things (there were none), I drew great comfort in knowing an entire department was pouring its resources into my singular case, consulting centers worldwide for insights on surgical techniques, passionately and excitedly embracing my crisis as if their careers depended on it. Little did I realize what a feather this could be in their caps. Good enough, for something had happened which raised the stakes even higher, yet gave me the greatest motivation to beat cancer that a person can know: we had been told earlier that same week that we were expecting. I was overjoyed, but could not show it, for fear the excitement would kill me.

Weeks turned into months as we waited for word of a surgery date. My doctor poured over case studies and traveled to observe similar operations to improve his ability to save my life. We busied ourselves with daily life as the months passed. Finally, my operation was scheduled — on the date our child was due! We said no. If I didn't survive the procedure, I would never have a chance to see my son, and I was determined to witness his entrance into this world. Of course, with the tumor becoming increasingly active as the months went by, it could be an embarrassing and unnecessary stress if I fainted in the delivery room. While I wouldn't be the first husband to have done that, I didn't want to be the first who died as a result.

Better to risk the joy of holding him, than to never hold him at all. I wondered if I could do it. I wondered if I would live to have a family. What kind of life would we share? And, if I didn't make it, would I be able to watch over him from the other side? Because these questions were too big and emotional to tackle, I concentrated instead on more immediate problems, like jumping the final hurdle on the road to graduation.

It was my final year of seminary. While no longer taking services, I was still experiencing considerable stress over my academic Achilles heel: Greek. We were required to learn at least one of the ancient languages in order to translate the scriptures directly. I had never been adept at this; languages were a puzzle, and my mind seized up at every exam. One would think, having failed Greek four times by my final year that something would have stuck besides my brain. Now, in a crammed summer course, I was praying for a miracle and pressing my nose to the books. Late nights spent parsing verbs and memorizing root words yielded no improvement. I used every trick I could think of: study groups, tapes played during sleep, renditions through limericks, song and dance in the empty library. Finally, my professor (ever patient, even more so given my health) suggested I forget the exam and simply meet with him in his office. He would work with me, one on one, until I demonstrated sufficient comprehension for a pass. This was the breakthrough — I had frozen up in the written tests, but orally I sailed through. (What a concept, to learn a language by speaking it!) He gave me a pass, a prayer, and a hug. I left confident that if I could survive Greek, I could surely survive this operation.

September rolled in, and with it the birth of our son. He was two weeks past due, emerging gloriously new and magnificent. I was astounded and grateful that the event caused me to forget myself. Instead of adrenaline taking my breath away, he did. I was left feeling peaceful, hopeful, open, and unafraid. Leaving the hospital in the early morning light, I felt a future full of possibilities and a deep sense that my life was only beginning. This was borne of a knowing I could not explain.

It was not until our son was six months old that we finally received the date to proceed with the operation. I savored fatherhood all the more, my heart breaking with joy as he laughed and smiled, my soul filling with love while quietly holding him during late-night feedings, his Buddha face gazing up at me in the moonlit nursery. But that peace eluded me the evening before the operation. Restless, I went for a long walk to be alone with my thoughts. Just as I felt I had worn myself out enough to sleep, I returned to find the hospital had called: the surgery was delayed another week! I would still be admitted, but instead of removing the tumor they would use medications to slowly lower my blood pressure from the norm of 110/70 to a fragile 50/30. This would give them more time to respond should the tumor release its noradrenalin. Otherwise, my pressure would leap to fatal levels and I would be gone.

I was shocked. Was this something they had remembered at the last minute? Why hadn't we known this before? What of all the months spent learning, preparing, training for this procedure? All confidence collapsed with that single call, and me with it. The room spun, vision blurred, and I crumpled to the floor. I recall my wife helping me to the couch, then to the bed, where I lay shaking until sleep's escape.

The next morning we quietly drove to the hospital. The weight of worry suffocated conversation. We entered the hospital room to find my medical team waiting. I stood with celebrity status before this small audience, feeling more like a fragile guinea pig, a prize patient about to be eviscerated and devoured by the eager appetite of science. Introductions, procedural explanations, and assurances were delivered with stressed smiles and pressed lab coats. It all felt terribly surreal. After they left, we pulled the privacy curtain about my bed like a cocoon, and gazed at the little boy who smiled and cooed, blissfully oblivious to the trials of life.

Two days later I awoke in the intensive care unit to the familiar pulse of machines and the fog of lifting anesthetic. The surgery was a success, the doctors were elated, and I felt like I'd been through a war. There had been a considerable release of catecholamines, especially noradrenalin, as predicted. The metabolites flooded my system, shooting my blood pressure skyward. It was touch-and-go for a bit as my stats danced wildly in response to medications that brought the pressure down too low, then others to bring it up again. My surgeon, clearly relieved it was over, explained how, in bypassing the femoral artery, they had to cut some nerves, which would leave my right leg a bit weak. Otherwise, everything went as expected.

I lay in the unit that night looking out through glass doors at the other patients, feeling my life, tuned to the fragile gift we take for granted. While I spent considerable recovery time in prayer, connecting to God's presence and love, an intensely more apprehensible manifestation of love pulled me back to health: down the hall, my family sat in exhausted relief, helping my son learn to stand in the hospital corridors. I joined him in that challenge; it was over a week before I was able to shuffle on my own. Slowly, carefully, I would rise, resting against a nurse, resting in a chair, and finally resting in the car, heading for home. I made it to graduation, and in a few months we moved to Lampman, Saskatchewan, a tiny town of six hundred people on the vast prairie. It was my first parish, where on my first day, a frail man died and I found myself sitting by a hospital bed once again. Little did I know this would be my heart's calling, and the most satisfying aspect of ministry I could imagine.

CHAPTER 7

THE WAY OF RECONCILIATION

Never does the human soul appear so strong as when it
foregoes revenge and dares to forgive an injury.
— EDWIN HUBBELL CHAPIN

ASK SOMEONE ABOUT THEIR LOVE, AND THEY WILL TELL YOU OF their loss. Ask of successes and you will hear failures. It seems we cannot help but see the unfinished within, all the more when time is short and we lament what has been put off through the years. Top on the list is the brokenness. Relationships are the fabric of our souls, the only clothes we wear to heaven, and they are always torn and tattered. Nobody leaves here completely clean; there are loose ends, unfinished conversations, broken bits of hope locked in the heart, waiting for forgiveness.

This is where true healing is waiting, for to forgive another is to set yourself free from the pain that has smothered joy, life, and connection (mostly that you have with yourself). I always thought cancer would wake people up to this central work of the soul, but we are a stubborn and confused species, unaware of how we cling to pain as part of our identity, unaware of the power of forgiveness to heal the heart.

How do you hold what you desire without adding desire to it? I have met many patients caught in this dilemma as they practice their positive affirmations, cultivate healing energy, manifest a better reality, and claim their healing. One in particular had done a great deal of work reconnecting with spirit and experiencing forgiveness. She was quite aware of the abuse and traumas of her past, the disappointments that compromised unconditional love, and her patterns of self-sabotage. She felt her cancer was the result of the psychic energy from these injuries. From diagnosis, she got to work with a vengeance to stamp out any residual "negative energy" held in her consciousness. One day, she pronounced that she had found herself in an amazing state of heightened awareness, joy, and love.

"I have forgiven my past, this cancer no longer serves my growth," she declared. Yet, still it remained.

What was she doing wrong? Well, first, the very notion that there was a way to do it "right" sabotaged the whole process. This is not a matter of starting the day with meditation, yoga, and hemp oil while saying the rosary and dropping some coins in the panhandler's cup on the way to work. This is a matter of digging into the shadowlands of the soul and unearthing the ugly, the broken, the parts of us that fight to remain unknown.

While all healing is first an act of forgiveness, sometimes suffering is the only path through which we are shattered, die, and then reborn. (Ultimately, every act of creation is first an act of destruction.) Since nobody fights like family, dying brings the homework of forgiveness out of the shadows. Brittle wounds long left smoldering flare to life. And when the black sheep appears on the scene, family tensions are ramped up as the wounds of relationships gape silently and awkwardly in the room.

How simply the bridge can be built. All it takes is a gesture, a nod, a tear, acknowledgment of the pain, permission to be broken and loved. It's a delicate move to invite someone to talk about his or her brokenness, but it is central to good spiritual care. I carefully watch a patient's body language as they hesitate on a story.

"Any regrets?" I might ask. Timed right, the tears will come, and the unfinished love story will flow. If this material is left unmet, the patient may become restless, depressed, picking at petty details and struggling through restless dreams. Death may be delayed until forgiveness is granted, upon which death comes more gracefully. The spirit is profoundly wise in the ways of reconciliation. Often a person will die on a birthday or anniversary, a mystical expression of solidarity and connection. I recall one case in which a palliative patient hung on for hours. Only after his estranged daughter spoke words of forgiveness and love did his death rattle cease. He left this world in peace. Yet there are many who have endured such cruelty that for them to forgive is a greater miracle than if their cancer had been cured.

PAST AND PRESENT TRAUMA

ACCORDING TO THE WORLD HEALTH ORGANIZATION, NORTH AMERICA HAS the lowest rate of violence against women, at 23 percent.[34] However, unreported cases lurk like the mass of an iceberg beneath the surface of civilized society. Sexual assault is the most under-reported crime because of fear and being commonly dismissed as marital tension.

This nightmare often extends back to childhood, and is the dark reality we never speak of: one in three girls, and one in seven boys, are sexually abused by the time they reach eighteen.[35] It is a global travesty, among humanity's greatest shames.

Awareness of abuse is critical in supporting these patients when faced with a cancer diagnosis, as present traumas naturally trigger past ones. How an abused person copes with an experience in which they feel overwhelmed, powerless, or scared will largely be determined by how they survived in the past. In this dynamic is both power to endure and potential for self-destruction, especially if the survival skills served the individual well, since those skills can be both positive coping strategies and maladaptive ones. These may include self-medicating and destructive behaviors, such as substance addiction. They were used to escape the psychological pain of abuse. They may resurface in the journey through cancer. The patient may also find dreams and memories of abuse are triggered, haunting them through treatment.

Survivors of abuse, like survivors of cancer, also tend to feel they survived for a reason. This makes being hit with cancer feel like an especially brutal blow. The capacity to endure may entail cutting off the emotional connection to one's vulnerability, one's fear, and one's humanity. The result is depersonalization, the severing of the psyche from the experience.

As if this wasn't hard enough, the situation is greatly compounded with breast, gynecological, and rectal cancers. Examinations and treatment can trigger somatic memories of abuse, leaving the patient trapped in a nightmare the clinician is oblivious to. Yet there are simple, basic things healthcare professionals can do: make screening for abuse a standard assessment question for all women with gynecological cancers and men with prostate cancer; have a healthcare provider compassionately explain any procedure; treat the person, not the anatomy; believe patients when they say a procedure is painful, and do something about it; ensure patients see the same doctor for all appointments and examinations (while clinically, this may seem impossible, it's worth changing the system to accommodate). Remember that some examinations and procedures can feel like an extreme violation, especially brachytherapy. This highly effective treatment involves the placement of radioactive material directly into a tumor. Often used for cervical and prostate cancer, it is critical to administer this with utmost sensitivity and care, especially if there is no sedation.

Survivors of abuse feel they must comply and endure pain and humiliation silently because it is a medical procedure. Although the treatment could be lifesaving, nurses report there are some patients who cannot continue due to psychological distress, even though they describe the therapists as very compassionate and respectful. Since the best care empowers the patient, giving her as much control as possible in this situation can only help: show her the instruments used, allow her power to stop when she is overwhelmed, have counselors available before and after, or arrange a peer support meeting with someone who's gone through it. Following these simple steps can prevent unnecessary trauma and provide wise, respectful care.

Even though sexual abuse is among the most brutal and degrading acts people are capable of, the power of the human spirit to not only endure but also to heal and forge meaning out of suffering is greater. Working wisely and compassionately with this devastating narrative can shift the internal balance of power from oppression to opportunity, to a new engagement with life and with one's self. Most do this work slowly, step by step, inching toward healing as they engage the fears and desperate places of the soul. And sometimes, impossibly, it happens all at once.

FORGIVENESS

AT FIFTY, LIZ WAS DEALING WITH BREAST CANCER AND A VIGOROUS CHE-motherapy that required hospitalization. A diminutive woman, one could tell nonetheless by the depth of her eyes that there was great power within her. Our introductory conversation quickly moved to heavier explorations on coping, suffering, and meaning. It was here that she shared an astonishing story: her cancer had become a catalyst, the instrument in healing a family rift stretching back eighteen years.

Almost two decades earlier, Liz had her father arrested for child abuse. He had sexually abused her, her sisters, and several children in the area. Now a convicted pedophile, this man had served fifteen years in prison. One would think that would be the beginning of the healing for their hearts: justice had been served, danger had been removed, and life could go on. For many victims of sexual abuse, though, a part of them never heals; instead, it gets repressed so the rest of them can move on.

Those children continued with their lives, trying to repair this primal injury, each in their own way escaping the terror. They employed suppression and depersonalization — strategies that enable endurance — but when his crimes were exposed, so were their wounds. Everyone felt the threat of them becoming fresh and open once again. They had left the past behind, and they didn't want to go back. To remember was to enter the nightmare again, to become possessed by the pain. His children also felt caught between two duties: to love their father, the provider, and to hate their foe, the abuser. Often, the instinctive, paternal obligation wins out. Liz couldn't let the past be the past, and she desired justice. So she had bravely brought it all into the present — all the pain, all the shame, and all the consequences. The result, for Liz, was rejection. Her family never spoke with her again.

Eighteen years later, she sat in a hospital room and received her cancer diagnosis. Composed and aware, she was able to absorb the information on treatment, side effects, possible outcomes, and probable death. Outside the room, her mother nervously paced the hall. She had good reason, for in her concern for what they knew would be cancer, she had contacted Liz's father. He sat in the waiting room a few doors down.

My gasp was audible as I listened to the story. Of all the times in Liz's life, this was not the one to have him present. It was the most vulnerable moment, the worst time to bring him back into her life; it felt to me a violation, an astonishingly cruel thing to do. It became, for Liz, the pivotal moment in which she could choose grievance or grace.

"There was this quiet knock on the door. I was just telling my mother the news, how I needed chemotherapy, how sick I could get. And there was this knock. I thought it was the nurse, so I said 'Come in', and there was my father. He slowly walked in and stood there, as close as you are to me. And I wasn't afraid. I wasn't angry. I didn't hate him. I just felt this peace. I felt compassion and peace, and I got up and hugged him, and he crumbled. He cried and collapsed in the chair. And I was good. I don't know how I did that. It wasn't me, it must have been God. But I'm at peace, and have never felt more … myself. Because of this, my sisters are talking to me again.… Well, all but one. She's still angry, but she's always been that way."

To be honest, I found I wanted to interrupt her story of reconciliation, to encourage her *not* to forgive, for when that happens prematurely it is not only unhealthy but also reinforces the victim's powerlessness. A wound healed over prematurely can fester. This is no less true with our heart. What drove her to instinctively release the pain she had felt all those years? Was it cancer that composed her character or was it really disengagement once again from her vulnerable self? I still don't know, but I suspected the former, because she related this with astonishing emotional insight. It was clear Liz did not want to be like her angry sister. That pain would not possess her anymore.

The first and often only person to be healed by forgiveness is the person who does the forgiving. Liz seemed to have set herself free. I found myself filled with admiration and astonishment at her strength, and told her so.

"Really?" was her reply. "Well, to me, I'm just me."

As is often the case, we cannot see ourselves from within our own experience, we can only look out. It's our "normal." Liz credits her cancer for this reconciliation. Cancer enabled her to forgive, which was an act of remembering and honoring her own dignity and that of her father, even if he failed to do that himself. Liz suspected, though, that he had learned this vital lesson, for he seemed to be deeply repentant, and carried himself with quiet humility, demonstrating new respect for the women in his life. I thought Liz was exceptional, and told her so: a person who overcame childhood trauma through the growth and insight provided by yet another traumatic crisis.

ABSOLUTION

HE WAS ALMOST NINETY, AND WEPT CONSTANTLY IN HIS ROOM. THE NURSE asked if I could help, for he would soon die, and as hard as they tried, he remained inconsolable. Once he realized I was a chaplain, the conversation turned to the core of his pain: he was terrified of God's judgment. Something unforgivable weighed him down. To my horror, it was child abuse, and he had been the perpetrator.

It had happened over sixty years earlier, a troubled time of addiction and hardship in which he spun with dark desires and cruelty. He had been caught and, rare for that time, was tried and found guilty. Fifteen years of prison almost destroyed him, but somehow life balanced out, brought him a vocation he loved, and the courage to express his regret over what he had done. Nonetheless, he remained alone through the years, never able to love or be loved as he needed. Now he lay on his deathbed, weeping. Even though I knew there are few things worse than to die with regret, feeling you have wasted or, worse, desecrated life, I found my own disgust and rage toward this man build into a loathing that almost blocked my ability to see his humanity, his brokenness.

It was only in the long silence after his confession that I was able to recognize the revulsion as my issue, to offer it to God and ask for His vision. A wave of pain and sorrow moved through me, and we sat in his tears. Then I quietly leaned forward and said the rite of confession and forgiveness. The words took on new weight....

"We confess we are in bondage to sin and cannot free ourselves. We have sinned against you in thought, word and deed, by what we have done, by what we have left undone. We have not loved you with our whole heart, we have not loved our neighbors as ourselves. For the sake of your Son, Jesus Christ, have mercy on us. Forgive us, renew us, and lead us, so that we may delight in your will and walk in your ways, to the glory of your son, Christ our Lord." Then the absolution, words of liberation, words of hope. "God forgives you all your sins. God forgives you."

What was I really saying? When we forgive, we choose to see the light and beauty in the other, even if he doesn't honor it in himself. We choose to see the other as a child of God, an immortal expression of Divine Love. We choose to no longer identify the other with his pain, or our own. We chose to remember: forgiveness is the key to peace.

He lay quietly for some time, eyes closed and tears streaming down his face. "Is the peace I feel from the medication, or is it real?" he quietly asked. I sat with him in silent prayer, my hand resting gently upon his. Late in the night, long after I left, he died peacefully in his sleep, a soft smile upon his face.

I have never encountered a soul completed before death. Nonetheless, from what I have witnessed, we can be confident that we will never be alone. Even when our spirit has been crushed by neglect and abuse, there is a work of love begun in us that will be seen through to its completion, if not in this life, then certainly in the next.

The journey back to our best self is universal. Derek Walcott writes of this in a poem called "Love After Love." It explores the universal pilgrimage through the labyrinth of relationships and the wounds of life; to arrive back at home (as all good pilgrimages do) in our own heart and to realize that what we were searching for all along was within us. The poem concludes by inviting us:

> Take down the love letters from the bookshelf,
> the photographs, the desperate notes,
> peel your own image from the mirror.
> Sit. Feast on your life.[36]

How do you feast on your life when it holds such horrors as sexual abuse? Even for those who have had a relatively smooth journey devoid of trauma, celebrating yourself stirs discomfort and unease. It feels selfish, it feels narcissistic. These labels reveal our effort to avoid the most difficult homework of our life: to love ourselves as God does. This is noble work; it is the hero's journey into the heart, where the shocking truth of our identity is waiting: that we are children of the Divine, manifestations of God's love and consciousness. What a contrast to the messages of the subconscious!

Just try this exercise for a moment: Close your eyes, and silently say, "Despite my (*fill in the blank here* … body, shortcomings, insecurities), I completely love and accept myself." Notice your reaction. If you are among the few who can own this with peace and gratitude, you are deeply blessed. It's so much easier to play small — less responsibility, less consequence, a more comfortable ride. But, oh, the treasure we miss!

Parker Palmer, founder of the Center for Courage and Renewal, comments on the root of this division within the self. "Afraid that our inner light will be extinguished or our inner darkness exposed, we hide our true identities from each other. In the process, we become separated from our own souls. We end up living divided lives, so far removed from the truth we hold within that we cannot know the integrity that comes from being what you are."[37]

This is true for all of us. This is why the agenda of life is not so much to be good as to be real. Since God is love, only love is, ultimately and eternally, real. So, no matter how hard we try to avoid it, that work of loving ourselves as God does will always be waiting. It is the work of authentic engagement. It cannot, fundamentally, be avoided.

CHAPTER 8

THE WISDOM OF GRIEF

There is no love of life without despair of life.

— ALBERT CAMUS

CRISES, LIKE CANCER, TEND TO DISTILL THE DOMINANT ASPECTS of a personality: a gentle person may become more compassionate; a controlling person may become more obsessive. At times, the disease and its treatment can reduce you to your most primitive components. Fear flares as anger, with healthcare staff and family receiving the brunt of it. Security becomes an illusion as you grasp to control breathing and bowels, pain and the promise of a better day. All the while, life is falling apart. Perhaps you're feeling worse on the medicine than you did from the cancer. Perhaps you're seeing the buried distress in your loved ones' eyes and shield the burden of love in your own as they care for you.

Yet, even while cancer may threaten to take your life, it also amplifies it with the message, *Look. Feel. Taste. Be aware. Don't miss this. Don't miss this beautiful, ordinary day. It may be the last time you feel this good, taste this food, take this step.* The critical homework of authentic engagement is before you. It is the bumpy road to full awareness. It is the training to be awake to the life you have and to love the people you're with. It turns out that very little of cancer is about the medicine. Grief is the heart of this homework, and you can't get to gratitude without it.

We are all experts in grief, and students of it as well. This visceral hit to the foundation of our being registers in the gut, sends the head spinning, collapses the lungs, and tears the heart with a palpable ache — the body knows it well. The mind, however, scrambles to lock it down and maintain control, which is why we repeatedly miss the wisdom of grief as a powerful opportunity to love more deeply. Grief is the price you pay for love, an insight the Lebanese-American artist and poet Khalil Gibran expressed beautifully:

> Your joy is your sorrow unmasked.
> And the selfsame well from which your laughter rises was
> oftentimes filled with your tears.[38]

Patients and families teach me this every day, with every mourning and every moment. Their lessons carve into my being, deepening my humanity and my resilience as one who can love through the loss.

This must be the hardest part of growing through cancer, and the lessons begin long before the disease appears. It starts the moment your first ice cream falls from the cone, the moment you lose your favorite blanket or toy. It continues with the loss of moving to a new community, seeing friendship fade, enduring and astonishingly surviving your first breakup. We lose our keys. We lose our hair. We lose our health. We lose our minds. Every loss is a rehearsal for the final loss, when we leave our loved ones, moving into that darkness, that all-knowing light. As we bear the loss of people, places, and objects, our identity (who we are in this world through our relationships) also changes. And this prepares us for the big ones: loss of health, job, vitality, independence, role as provider or caregiver, loss of our faculties, consciousness, and finally our body. With that, everything we have ever known as real and every relationship we've ever had is on the table as we fold our hand.

What a wonderful surprise to find that the love we've known with others is actually eternal. Since God is love, our connection with those we love must also be eternal — the one thing we take with us.

ROBERT

THE BEST PART OF LIFE IS THE ABILITY TO SHARE IT, WHICH MAKES THE worst thing about cancer not what it does to you, but what it does to those you love.

Robert's wife was dying. While she knew it and was able to talk about it plainly with me, being so transparent with Robert was another matter. She described him as the rock, always able to keep it together, always the calm in the storm. She asked if I could break through to his pain. Her heart craved to share an intimate vulnerability with him. The disconnection of his "strength" was a greater heartache than dying itself.

Knowing his smile was a mask to stave off despair, I looked to create a safe space where he could remove it. That came one day in the hall. Pleasantries marked our pace to privacy, where he could honestly encounter himself. It's so helpful to have an office by the elevators. An open door gently invites lives and stories in — lives that want to feel safe and connected, stories that contain ultimate hopes and fears.

"I notice Karen will talk openly with me about dying, but she holds you carefully on that shifting ground," I offered. "She protects you. And in our conversations, you speak of her dying, but won't mention it with her. You are both so careful, but it creates a disconnection. Here it is, the most heart-wrenching and significant event ever to occur, and you hide from each other, from yourselves. Your love for each other is so beautiful, but your conversation is like a hesitant lament."

This is often the case. There's so much grief waiting to be expressed, but we protect each other from that distress. As a result, no one is able to be authentically present and connected; yet, that is our heart's desire, to be so loved that we feel safe, to be so loving that we feel courage. This cannot be experienced unless we are authentically present in the mess.

I wanted to get deep into Robert's pain without triggering his defense mechanisms. A good way to do this was to reflect off his nobility, his love, honoring both his and his wife's dignity in the struggle. "I know a bit of your story with each other. I know you two have been through many ups and downs. Yet your love has been deep and constant, and you carry yourself with a profound grace, even as you see her dying. I'm wondering what that does to you."

We sat in silence. He began to tear up. At this moment, the instinct may be to rescue the other person from their distress, to reach out and comfort. But the best work in this conversation happens in the silent spaces. Robert began to collapse, to disintegrate, which was perfect, for here there was no need to hide. Here was his raw pain; here, he would be naked to himself. Silence was the catalyst for confession, wherein he could come back to himself, to the one he had ignored for another. And he began to share, through his tears, how he couldn't imagine life without her. The anticipatory grief became the actualized grief, no longer cloaked. He was so scared it would destroy him, yet grief brought him back to himself, and because of that, more authentically to her. They experienced a new level of intimacy in those final days, more in love than ever before. And Robert was so grateful, in the end, to discover his vulnerability was the greatest gift he could give her.

ANTICIPATORY GRIEF

WHILE YOU MAY BE FAMILIAR WITH THE PHASES OF GRIEF DEVELOPED BY Elisabeth Kübler-Ross, I have found they are never linear. They are lumpy, messy, and confusing. So, instead of analyzing denial, anger, depression, bargaining, and acceptance, I'd like to simply look at the two sides of grief, from the perspective of those losing and from the one leaving.

Loved ones go through **anticipatory grief**, preparing to lose that person they cannot bear to lose. This is not conventional grief begun early; this is a silent rehearsal of the inevitable. It doesn't reduce the intensity of grief afterwards, but studies show it can reduce the duration.[39]

Anticipatory grief can leave family members feeling guilty, as if they are giving up hope and abandoning the patient. Know that as long as you are there for support, you are doing all you can. When treatments fail, when cancer spreads with a vengeance, when you find yourself in an ICU staring down at your loved one ... these are the times when you (sometimes secretly) accept that the illness is terminal. Recovery is no longer a possibility. Focus on what you are doing — still supporting, still caring, still loving, and still creating meaningful moments together. You are shifting your energy from hope for recovery to hope for meaningful connection. You are ensuring the dying patient is not alone. It will break your heart and be the greatest privilege in the world.

Derek Thompson writes of this in his essay "The Secret Life of Grief." His words will be more eloquent than mine:

> My mom died on July 18, 2013, of pancreatic cancer, a subtle blade that slips into the host so imperceptibly that by the time a presence is felt, it is almost always too late. Living about 16 months after her diagnosis, she was "lucky," at least by the new standards of the parallel universe of cancer world. We were all lucky and unlucky in this way. Having time to watch a loved one die is a gift that takes more than it gives.
>
> Psychologists call this drawn out period "anticipatory grief." Anticipating a loved one's death is considered normal and healthy, but realistically, the only way to prepare for a death is to imagine it. I could not stop imagining it. I spent a year and a half writing my mother a goodbye letter in my head, where, in the private theater of my thoughts, she died a hundred times.[40]

Anticipatory grief is not simply normal grief you prepare for. It's so much more, containing many losses: changing roles in the family, financial challenges, increasing responsibilities as you think about being a single parent, loss of the dreams of what could be. One grieves possible futures, as well as lamenting the past that cannot continue.

So what can you do? Be compassionately aware. When we know death is imminent, our bodies are often in a state of hyper-alertness; we panic whenever the phone rings, when an email arrives, when breathing changes. This can become mentally and physically exhausting. Acknowledge the profound emotional toll this takes on you.

When death eventually comes, there may be a residue of guilt for feeling relief. This is common and completely normal. It does not diminish your love for that person but speaks to the emotional load you've been carrying and acknowledges the release of that chapter of life. Derek Thompson expresses this beautifully in his same article: "In the weeks after she died, something strange happened. I did not plunge. Life did not stop. Instead, I felt something so unspeakably strange, so blasphemous, that I wondered if I could talk or write about it, at all. I felt okay."[41]

We are wired for equilibrium, and if other aspects of life are fairly good — relationships, sense of purpose, depth of love — then you will find balance again. Trust that your grief is wise and honors the relationship. Be real with it; be authentically human in it, so you can be transformed by it.

Preparatory Grief

WHILE OTHERS ANTICIPATE THE PATIENT'S DEATH, THE ONE DYING PRE-pares for it. The depth of that grief is markedly different, for while we get ready to say goodbye to one person, the dying prepare to say goodbye to everyone, to everything. As ultimate as that grief is, it can often be boiled down to four things: concern for loved ones, fear of suffering, unfinished business, and actual death.

Because grief is the price we pay for love, worry for loved ones becomes the primary concern. Patients ruminate on how their death will weigh upon others. They may feel guilt for being "a burden," the cause of existential suffering. This is an expression of both powerlessness and compassion, often causing the patient to protect their family from the reality of a poor prognosis or the truth of how suffering is experienced. Meanwhile, the family is protecting the patient from openly contemplating death in order to spare emotional pain. However, it is precisely that grief which becomes a bridge to belonging. Here you are, fighting for more moments of life, but avoiding the moment you have because it feels too overwhelming. You dare not allow others to see how you are shattered, for that would break open the floodgates; it would all come pouring out. The one you're truly protecting, in this case, is yourself. What if the most beautiful gift you can give your loved ones is their own pain? It is theirs to experience as part of their love, and as you hold them back from that, you delay the important work of authenticity that is aching to be realized.

Fear of suffering is the second concern (as long as physical suffering is not out of control). When medications are balanced, when a nurturing environment enables the dying person to feel the compassion of others, then they are freed to wrestle with the emotional and spiritual material of life. The body, unfortunately, can endure far more than we give it credit for, so it is critical to be aware of the signs of suffering before they get out of hand. These include fever, weakness, nausea, change in cognition, and of course, physical pain. Keeping ahead of this last one is best done by taking pain medications regularly, before it escalates to an unmanageable level. Some patients do this poorly, under-reporting their pain when asked, feeling they should be able to manage it on their own. Others fear becoming addicted, so are reluctant to take any medications. Sharing these concerns with the healthcare team is the best way to manage the pain wisely.

Suffering is so much more than a physical issue. Spiritual suffering, or existential distress, can dominate the mind, debilitate the soul, and be present even with treatable cancers. Our imagination can be more painful than the cancer.

This was the case with one woman who, after diagnosis, couldn't sleep, couldn't get the fear of death out of her head, even though she was diagnosed with a cancer that responds well to treatment, and she could have a normal lifespan. Because she had never spent a day in a hospital as a patient, but had spent many as a supportive daughter to her mother who had died of cancer, the only reference she had was her mother's suffering, her mother's deterioration, her mother's death. Now she was living the nightmare of walking in her mother's shoes. How to deal with this?

First, I named the thought of death for her. "You've been thinking of this from the moment you were diagnosed, and your mom is the only experience you've had. You're terrified that you're walking the same road as her."

"Yes!" was the immediate response, exclaimed with relief, as she experienced someone seeing her, acknowledging her pain and fear.

We begin this work by checking our perspective: Is the cancer life-threatening? What are the dangers of treatment? What are the triggers in this experience? Often, those include a loved one's death, unfinished business, and, most of all, the impact on those you love. Remember, the number one concern of people facing a serious illness is not their own fate, but the well-being of those they care for.

If death is a probable outcome, even if it won't happen for a year or more, we still name it. Run the hypothetical. What's your greatest fear, besides the well-being of your loved ones? Suffering. So, what can we do to alleviate that? Knowledge is power (or at least, the comforting illusion of power — we'll take what we can get!). How does one die of this type of cancer? Where would you want to be as you die? While many people answer "at home," others do not want the memory of their death in the home to taint or imprint upon their family. This is a way of protecting their loved ones. If in the home, what's needed? (Pain control, nursing support, having a bed located with easy access to an exit and to a bathroom.) Though most want to die at home, the majority die in hospital, where they are assured of twenty-four-hour nursing care, excellent pain management, and medical support. Often, a middle ground is the most comforting option: staying at home as long as possible and coming into hospital when needed. Discussing this can bring great comfort and relief from the fear of dying, and from the affliction of imagined outcomes. The earlier this conversation happens in the course of your illness, the sooner you will be able to normalize your fears and work wisely with distress.

Addressing the third concern, unfinished business, is where much of my work is done. No life leaves this world complete; however, it is possible to release what is left undone to the grace of God, trusting that even the tattered ends of your story are redemptive and enough. Exploring this is best done with genuine curiosity about your journey. As you look back, what were your life lessons that stand out? Most importantly, what is your unfinished love story? Here we allow lament to have a voice. It always feels easier to name our incompleteness than honor our accomplishments. As we explored in the previous chapter, these wounds become beautiful threads in the human story when redeemed through forgiveness.

What lies beyond death is the fourth concern, perhaps because it's so far beyond our scope of comprehension. Death, for many, is like a black hole; it swallows everything, and beyond the event horizon, it's all mystery. The closest we can imagine is sleep, yet that only opens the fear of being trapped in an illusionary world. What if it's a nightmare? What if it's chaos? Hamlet's words become our foreboding: "To sleep, perchance to dream — ay, there's the rub."[42] If you are, or have been a patient, then you know how we avoid this aspect of preparatory grief by putting emotional resources into what needs to be done here and now, in the waking hours. But at night … at night it's different. The hospital corridors are quiet, the darkness mutes distractions, and you are left with your own thoughts. That's when you have the space, away from other people's energy and anxiety, to contemplate where, or what, or how, or if you will be at all beyond this physical plane. So huge is this question that many people end up leaving the mystery to take care of itself.

"I don't have the answer," one patient related to me. "But I think the answer has me." This is the heart's hope; that the promise of the afterlife is waiting, that the grace of God will receive us.

Those with deep faith tend to approach the afterlife with confidence and expectation. However, there are studies that indicate the more controlling and conservative the religious tradition, the greater the existential anxiety as death approaches.[43] An image of a judgmental God, the fear of hell, leaves a residue of concern, which reinforces one's sense of unworthiness. I have witnessed more than a few of the faithful (from many traditions) enter those final days with their fingers crossed. It's a privilege to assure them that God's love is greater than we can comprehend, and though death will take them from this world, God will take them from death, and give them new life.

But all of that is in the future. What occupies a person's heart in a health crisis tends to be the reality they do know — here and now. Which is why preparatory grief doesn't wait until things get bad; it begins at the moment of diagnosis, and then undulates in a dark dance through the course of illness. This negotiation with mortality is core homework for the human soul and moves at an accelerated pace in the patient, compared to the anticipatory grief of the family.

I recall wrestling with this in my cancer journey. I was aware that many with my type of tumor die from a cardiac episode, and while five years' survival is good for those who have the tumor removed, the greatest risk of dying is when surgeons are removing it. Every time I've gone in for an operation, I've wondered where I would wake up, "here" or "there."

In the first two experiences, I prepared the way any naive young man would prepare: by brushing it off, acting like I had it all together. When I married and had a child, it was harder. I had so much more to lose. Though my preparatory grief was exponentially greater, I never spoke of it. When asked how I was doing, I would respond with the universal words of dismissal and deflection: "Oh, I'm fine." But "F-I-N-E" really meant Flustered, Insecure, Neurotic, and Emotional. It's a mask, because all our lives we are pushing against death. All our distractions and indulgences are ways to mediate that finality. Yet, cancer also taught me not to negotiate anymore, but simply to try to live life well. You would think having had four tumors would make me a master of that, but I'm as inconsistent as the next person. (In fact, I would say thicker than most. If there's a spiritual lesson behind cancer, it took me four rounds to finally get it!) While certainly not enlightened, I know I am very lucky to be here. Most days, that's more than enough.

No one moves through this smoothly; there are countless opportunities to trip and stumble over yourself. First there's the shock of diagnosis, which numbs comprehension and stifles hearing. Chaos condenses in your heart as you try to maintain normal life with the fresh awareness of what has always been there — your mortality. Fired by imagination, distress builds and is repeatedly dismissed with the distractions of daily life. Because preparatory grief is erratically experienced, there are moments when you can't contain it, yet in sharing it with others, you end up dealing with their anxiety as well! Immediately, it registers on their faces — that ashen, flat look. Eyes avert yours, and then they share their story, some family member who overcame, or worse, "succumbed" to the disease. Though you feel their disconnection, you hold your tongue. You know, though, that it's not the same. It's never the same. All experiences are individual experiences, and woundedness is holy ground. The least others can do is take off their shoes.

What people say to comfort can cause a surprising, secret reaction within the one with cancer. We hide it to protect the other, to maintain the peace, to abide by social rules. That reaction is anger. Why? Because the effort to honor another's pain becomes an insult toward it when not backed by full and even aching empathy. Otherwise, it feels like a kind but awkward foray into our vulnerability. And we respond with a smile. We say thank you, or even comfort them with an edited version of our reality that soothes their incomplete sincerity. "I'm doing fine." "It's not so bad, actually." "Yes, I've had better days."

I know it's hard. In the casual encounter we often lack the imagination and quality of presence to be anything more than two dimensional. What a gift it is to meet a supportive soul who listens through their entire being, not just their ears. They extend themselves naturally into our experience and hear the resonance of sorrow and fear. And they do not shrink back, or run away. They wait. Their silence creates a space in which we can emerge from the shadow of strength. Their ability to hold the awkward moment with tenderness makes it feel safe to be vulnerable, afraid, unsure, and human.

Then there's the person who really is trying to be supportive, but drops the ball. "You don't look sick!" (Thanks. You've just confirmed that you don't really understand what I'm going through.) "Live in the moment. Be strong. Attitude is everything." (These all imply that I'm not strong, I'm doing it wrong.) "Believe in miracles." (Is it that hopeless?) "If anyone can beat this, you can." (You really don't know how scared I am, do you?)

"It could be worse." (This is something only the patient can say, not the observer.) "It's part of a larger plan." "Everything happens for a reason." (Then sign me up for a different plan.) "This is your opportunity to deal with all that negative energy you've been suppressing." (And who are you to judge? Why don't you have cancer, then?) "I thought chemo was supposed to make you lose weight." (Someone should just slap you.) Worse, you end up being stalked by some optimist who buys pink pajamas and sends daily inspirational quotes. Please!

Grief is not something to be fixed; it is something to be processed. There's no use minimizing it or protecting the patient, though that may be the family's instinct. They will understandably be concerned about their loved one's feelings on death but will rarely ask about them, for to do so is more than they feel able to handle. In confronting the hard homework of truly wrestling with oblivion — the end of all that was and is known — what patients truly desire is a companion in the journey, not an assurance of the arrival.

This is why I am sometimes blunt. "What do you think the moment of death is like? Who would you like to be here as you die? Would you like to be awake or asleep? Would you like any music playing? Are there any rituals or conversations you need to happen? What is left unfinished? How can you let that go? What needs to be forgiven?" And, most importantly, "Tell me about the love." Be prepared for some deep conversation, and bring tissue.[44]

Most people, if they are aware in those last minutes, are actually not afraid to die. Instead, they feel an amazing peace come upon them.[45] There is a release of life, of time, of hopes. There is melancholy reflection, but more than that, a desire for others to know they were loved. This is expressed with profound gratitude. The patients I have had the privilege of supporting, who were aware to the end, have been great teachers in love and release.

If the patient is unconscious, I work with the families, assuming the patient can hear us nonetheless. Getting families to connect to their hearts, so the tears and stories flow, is a wonderful way to ensure the death is transformative, not simply traumatic.

The nuances around anticipatory and preparatory grief are far-reaching. There are so many attendant feelings and memories, all part of the intricate tapestry of our lives. Underneath there is always one theme: love. How have I loved? From that comes guilt, if we feel we have not loved well; anger, as a defense against guilt; or regret, for there will be no more opportunities to love. Fortunately, there can also be a surprising and graceful peace, gratitude that swells the heart and brings the tears, and most unexpected of all, freedom. This freedom emerges from the acceptance of what is. No longer resisting the reality of dying, one's energies are liberated from protecting others and yourself. A lightness of being comes upon you by being fully present in the moment — no expectations, no trying to be other than how you are. No longer straining for more moments of life, you discover that this one holds you. And this, of course, is the natural state of spirit, which is never anywhere else than here, now.

In the background, in the heart of at least one family member, will be the hope for a miracle. This is rarely an expression of faith but more often one of fear, anxiety, and helplessness. Instead of correcting this desperate plea for love and life to continue, I ask, "What would a miracle look like for you?" Often the response will be, "Well, I'd like the chemo to work. I'd like my child to live. I'd like there to be a cure." Understandable, but in the face of death is a greater miracle waiting: the capacity to love and endure and stay with pain and suffering, to be the love and light you are looking for.

It's hard. It's so hard. Grief is a thread knotted to all the losses of our lives, and we feel so powerless within it. Yet, it is at these times that we connect to the greatest power within us, one that cannot come unless we know our brokenness.

CHAPTER 9

WORKING WITH THE MIND

You are the sky. Everything else — it's just the weather.

— PEMA CHÖDRÖN

VULNERABILITY AND COURAGE

DISTRESS IS THE ADMISSION PRICE TO THE PRESENT MOMENT, FOR it reveals areas of our psyche that are unloved. The wisest response to distress is compassion: the ability to be present without attachment to any outcome. Being open to the catastrophe, you can use compassion as a keel to right yourself. It's an amazing and gentle skill to completely show up in the present moment, open to the emotional material we try so hard to hold in check — the wounds of childhood, the messages that say we have not loved well or been worthy of love. After all, the love we fail to give in life becomes the pain we carry through it.

No wonder we spend most of our energy avoiding ourselves. What an irony, taking chemotherapy or radiation to fight for more moments of life, yet to avoid the moment we are in. This disease that threatens to take our days also amplifies the gift of them and insists we pay attention. But how can we do that without falling apart? The key seems a contradiction: to be both vulnerable and strong.

Vulnerability and courage. The two go hand in hand. Brené Brown, points out in her TED Talk that "courage," comes from the Latin *cor*, meaning "heart," and the word originally meant to be able to tell your story with your whole heart, with total honesty.[46] This is different from bravery, the capacity to continue when you are afraid. Courage enables us to be kind to ourselves first, and that enables us to be compassionate with others. Courageous, vulnerable people believe that what made them vulnerable also made them beautiful. Vulnerability is necessary for there to be deep, authentic humanity.

Vulnerability is connected to shame. The more vulnerable we feel, the less we want to talk about it. Yet Brown discovered that those who have a wholehearted sense of worthiness, a strong sense of love and belonging, are able to be both vulnerable and strong at the same time. They are able to share this. Why? Because they believe they are worthy of love. This enables them to stand compassionately in the midst of their "weakness" and be authentic. In doing so, others perceive them not as weak but as incredibly, beautifully courageous. This is the goal at the end of life: not to be good, or to have it all together, but to be real. No self-deception. No need to hide from what is within. No need to suppress the truth of your experience. Brené Brown remarks, "Not only is vulnerability the core of shame and fear and struggle for worthiness, but it's also the birthplace of joy, and creativity, of belonging, of love."[47]

Three Minutes

An exercise came to me that facilitates the tuning of our souls toward love. I don't recall if I thought of it, though it is so simple and naively optimistic that it likely came from me; however, I have seen it work so powerfully in even the most wounded individuals that I can only believe I inherited it from someone much wiser. Nonetheless, it is in my spiritual tool kit along with compassion, presence, vulnerability, meditation, sacraments, prayer, Therapeutic Touch, and counseling.

I introduce this with a warning: you will find this excruciating but only for a short while. Do this with someone you trust, because you're going to be working with your vulnerability.

Set a timer to three minutes, sit and hold hands (that's optional), gaze into each other's eyes, and say nothing. During the three minutes, you are to be aware of everything that arises within you. Listen for the feelings that bubble and swirl. Locate them within your body. Feel their edges and how they have current, depth, and energy like flowing water. Be able to name the swirl of feelings. Be aware also of the thoughts that jump and dance in your head, leading you down paths and inviting you to attach to imagined streams and realities. Let all this happen, and stay with it!

Your assignment is to use the other person as an amplifier, to turn up the volume on your own noise, yet not abandon any aspect of your experience, no matter how emotional or painful, no matter how wonderful or intoxicating. (Yes, it can go in that direction, especially if you're sitting with someone you love and are grateful for.) Tears may well up, smiles may burst out, and giggles may percolate around controlled anxiety. Let it all happen, ride the wave of your experience, so that you may develop, over time, greater awareness of your own presence.

We are exercising the discipline of mindfulness so that you don't miss any moments of life. Even the ordinary ones are saturated with beauty. And the dark ones, they are saturated with more than growth. They are the doorways to your deepest and greatest potential, they are the avenues and detours on the road to self-awareness, and you can't go down those routes without becoming uncomfortable. A bad day for your ego is a great day for your soul. That's why this is best done with compassion and curiosity. Yes, the critical voice is guaranteed to butt in. Yes, you will edit, judge, and filter your thoughts and feelings, pouring yourself through the sieve of expectation. We all do this, so simply be aware of its happening.

I was so self-conscious the first time I did this! I worried about my crooked nose and then fixated on my partner's wrinkles. It took some practice to ease into what is unnatural in our culture: to stare into another's eyes. It can be perceived as downright rude, inappropriate, or even threatening. It's a daring move to hold one's gaze. In humans and animals alike, this is either a prelude to attack or seduction; either way, you are consumed. So, take a deep breath while these ancestral instincts raise your blood pressure.

Notice the urge to look away, and if you do, simply reset the timer, recompose, and reconnect with your body. Breathe into it all. About the two-minute mark, you may find a shift in the quality of your presence. You may forget yourself in the other's eyes (always a beautiful experience), you may notice aches and pains, or you may want to run away. If that's the case, good — all the more material to work with! When the timer goes off, you can do whatever you want: grab a coffee, take a deep breath, cry and embrace, laugh like a child, or dash for the door. But I hope you will talk about it. Share how you shifted through that brief eternity. Train together every day (preferably when nothing else is pressing for your attention). And be excited about it, because you are learning how to connect with the most important person you could ever come to love — yourself.

Perhaps you don't have anyone to train with. One person asked me if she could do this with her cat. "No," I said. "You're guaranteed to lose that contest." (Yes, it does become a contest with a cat; they are superior in both the clarity of their intention and the consistency of their indifference to us. Dogs? They will have you grinning foolishly with licks and love so persuasive you'll happily remain on the surface where it's comfortable. Stick with your own species for this exercise. You can involve the four-legged varieties in the next one.) Even if you have no one available, you can still do this in a mirror. As three minutes tick by, you may find yourself gazing into a stranger's face. You may notice your pores, your wrinkles, and all the lovely imperfections that speak of your experience but make you reach for a mask. But we are here to take the mask off, so hold the gaze and listen with awareness and curiosity to all that arises within.

Interesting things happen when you compassionately show up to yourself. First, your distress rises. Then, with practice, it quickly shifts. You are changing the relationship to your own experience simply through the quality of your presence. By fully showing up, you are no longer straining against any aspect of yourself and are able to be someone more wonderful than a person who is keeping it all together: you are becoming more authentic. More real. More loving. This is a theme you will encounter often in this book because it is, I suspect, the greatest goal of our spiritual journey.

It's also good for your immune system. A Harvard study on Mindfulness for Persons with Cancer and Terminal Illness found that simple compassionate exercises increased immune system proteins, lowered cortisol levels, and improved sleep.[48] Never think there is nothing you can do.

BECOMING A WARRIOR

YOU ARE BECOMING WHAT IS KNOWN IN BUDDHISM AS A "BODHISATTVA," a warrior of compassion. I love this term, infused with both courage and vulnerability. It is the awakened mind, able to wholeheartedly stay with pain, suffering, anger, death, and not retaliate, judge, or change the outward circumstances. It is through softness and openness of presence that bodhisattvas transform the energy of limitation and despair. "Strong back, soft front" is their motto.

A story illustrates this. Once, there was a village overrun by a brutal warlord. In the modest temple at the center of the town, a monk sat in meditation. Suddenly, the doors burst open and a warrior charged in, screaming. The monk sat motionless and met the fiery gaze with a calm expression.

This caused the warrior to pause, then to scream, "Do you know who I am? I am one who can run you through with my sword without flinching!"

And the monk, after a pause, said with calm resolve, "Do you know who I am? I am one who can be run through with your sword without flinching."

You may be thinking, "What good is this practice if the monk gets run through, anyway?" It's important to realize that you are both the monk and the warrior. Time and time again, we let the enraged, fearful side of us slaughter the vulnerable, noble side. The critical mind of reactivity and control is quick to take up the sword in defense of the ego (who we think we are, the role we play without knowing it). That fearful, desperate side of us will cling to life as we knew it, even after that life is radically changed.

This practice is powerfully fulfilled in the life of Jesus, who responded to the suffering around him with profound compassion, who reacted to the betrayal of his friends and the brutality of his executioners with calm, loving awareness. The clarity of his connection to God provided an unshakable foundation from which he could encounter any experience as a true bodhisattva warrior. We see it in the Qur'an, which describes Allah as the Compassionate One. No other adjective is used so frequently to describe God in the Islamic text.[49] We see compassion in Judaism, in the central ethical mandate of *tikkun olam*, which means to repair the world. This Mishnah calls one to help beyond what is required, for in doing so, you restore a piece of the shattered divine spark. You are actually helping a wounded member of humanity remember their inherent dignity. You are honoring the light within them, even when they do not honor it themselves. What a transformation our world would undergo if we were to begin this sacred work, whatever our traditions or beliefs, by first honoring the sacredness of ourselves. This was the homework of one patient who discovered, through a single sentence, how he could guide his heart in the path to becoming a warrior of compassion.

MIKE

MIKE HAD JUST COMPLETED TREATMENT FOR PROSTATE CANCER. A DIVORCE and estrangement from his children marked the prelude to his diagnosis, and now, after a successful course of radiation and surgery, he was struggling with ongoing fatigue and unrealistic expectations of himself. The gift of life he had fought for was turning out to be a test of endurance against fates that conspired to destroy every good thing he had ever known. His sexual functioning had been drastically affected by the procedures as well (erections often are no longer possible after prostate surgery). He spent the days sleeping and the evenings drinking. He had lost himself as well as those he loved.

I asked him what he wanted from our conversations and what he wanted from life. His answer was poignant: "I want to come back to myself, to the man I know I can be. I don't want to spiral into a dark place of bitterness and regret. I want to be happy again."

We first discussed his attachments, including the attachment to that goal. Happiness is a byproduct of being authentic in relationships, starting with the relationship you have with yourself. His struggles were numerous, and I was only able to see him for short-term therapy. How could we awaken compassion in such a short time against such challenges? He needed a tool, and it needed to be a simple one. I paused before speaking, praying silently for the words to come. "I'm going to give you a sentence I want you to say before you take any action, whether that be making yourself a meal, or going to work, or calling your children. Say this silently to yourself as a meditation, and let it guide you in all your decisions, all your thoughts and perceptions. If you are being true to this sentence, then you will feel it in your heart as a growing peace and agreement. Your thoughts, words, and actions will align. If you are not being true to this sentence, then you will instinctively know that, too. Part of you will resist, rationalize, and react to it. Say this sentence with your heart, with your body, as well as your mind. Here is the sentence: 'This is how I love.'"

Mike sat silently as he rolled the words over in his mind. An eyebrow raised, he repeated the words, but interestingly, shifted them, revealing the instinctive resistance we all have to empowerment: "How should I love?"

"Notice what happened there?" I asked with excitement. "Did you see what happened? You changed it from an affirmation to an inquiry. All the power disappears. Say it out loud, 'This is how I love.' You're rising in the morning, 'This is how I love.' You're making yourself breakfast, 'This is how I love.' You're talking to your kids, 'This is how I love.' You're grieving your divorce, and feeling alone and frustrated, reaching for a drink, 'This is how I love.' What happens when you say it, silently in your heart? Feel the truth of it, and if love is not there, let it guide you to choose in ways that make it so."

Mike began to cry. He began to sob and crumple in the chair. "But I don't! I don't love! I fight and control and do anything I can not to be afraid." He cried with a release of pain he had defended for months. With that sentence, Mike compassionately opened to the wounded part of himself, and his healing journey began. It was not a journey he could do alone, so I connected him to Alcoholics Anonymous, he accessed a cancer support program, and most importantly, he reconciled with his children. We never discussed religion, faith, or God, yet we both knew he was on the way to healing his soul. Bodhisattva, Christ consciousness, *tikkun olam*, the Compassionate One. A small part of the world being restored.

ATTACHMENT AND LOSS

BUDDHIST NUN PEMA CHÖDRÖN MAKES HER HOME, I AM FORTUNATE TO say, just a few hours from mine, at Gampo Abbey, in Cape Breton, Nova Scotia. With humor and insight, she helps people explore how every loss is a challenge as to who we think we are and who we actually are. Every loss is a lesson in *shenpa*, a Tibetan term that means attachment. More accurately, it means "that which has its hooks in you." As she explains, this internal hook is felt most acutely when our buttons are pushed: "Somebody says a mean word to you and then something in you tightens — that's the *shenpa*. Then it starts to spiral into low self-esteem, or blaming them, or anger at them, denigrating yourself. And maybe if you have strong addictions, you just go right for your addiction to cover over the bad feeling that arose when that person said that mean word to you. This is a mean word that gets you, hooks you. Another mean word may not affect you but we're talking about where it touches that sore place — that's a *shenpa*."[50]

You know the feeling, the sudden emotion that chokes your coping and composure. It's the desperate urge to change the topic, to run from an abrupt sense of groundlessness and unease. *Shenpa* leaves you disoriented when you unexpectedly run into an old lover, when your wife or boss or friend says something that strikes a nerve, when you have the carpet ripped out from under you through a diagnosis.

You also know the reaction: the instinct to flee from it, fix it, or medicate it. Our escape plans are habitual: alcohol, food, sex, cigarettes, defensiveness, hostility, withdrawal, sleepiness, inappropriate behavior, giddiness, even telltale speech patterns and voice tones. Often our senses become blunted or exaggerated in an attempt to filter what we are experiencing. The classic example is receiving bad news. I recall one family member who became more cheery and attentive to everyone's needs, as if hosting a party, whenever the reality of the patient's suffering was addressed. She clearly was uncomfortable and unable to handle the complex emotions she was feeling. This was her way of protecting herself, but it was also how her emotional pain was controlling her.

Understanding why we react in such a way can help to temper our distressing feelings and behavior, to bring them under control through working with our own thoughts with compassion and awareness. We don't have to believe everything we think. We don't have to become victims. Identifying with the accusations is the attachment. What we must strive for is non-attachment, to distance ourselves from a knee-jerk reaction when we feel provoked or overwhelmed, in order to make a more balanced assessment. Emotions are part of human nature and, to a large extent, dictate our choices. The challenge is to identify the rogue reaction and to use its energy to return to a compassionate stance.

Curiosity is a wonderful tool when dealing with *shenpa*. With curiosity we can notice our anger, our joy, our grief, and ask, What's this about? What does this tell me about what I value, what I feel I am to lose or gain about who I think I am? What does this say about my life? Through curiosity we can dance with anger, grief, even death, and realize that, through this inquiry, we are stepping back from the experience rather than identifying with it. We are practicing a second Buddhist approach to suffering: *vipassana*, which means "to witness." In this meditation, one moves into the experience of attachment and suffering with the mantra, I have this body, but I am not this body. I have this thought, but I am not this thought. I have this feeling, but I am not this feeling. I am the witness.

I use this myself, for the intensity of my work will often trigger my own tears. It reminds me of the shortest passage in the Gospels, one that demonstrates a model of vulnerability and strength. It's from John 11:35, in which Christ comes to the grave of his friend Lazarus. It simply says, "Jesus wept." When I feel that rise in me, instead of suppressing it, I breathe into it as solidarity with the other person. To abandon any part of your own experience is to pull away from what is. Counselors must be present to the nuances of their own distress and move with the current of it.

Besides, supporting a person's grief without thinking it's going to affect you is like moving through water thinking you won't get wet. Identifying with another's distress is both the affliction of compassion and its greatest gift.

Who'd have thought such a simple tool could reveal that you are more than your mind. While the practice certainly helps me be fully present with suffering, I always marvel how *vipassana* brings patients back to their essential core and enables them to go beyond surviving, even to use cancer for the acceleration of their spiritual journey.

Chapter 10

REMARKABLE SURVIVORS

If you don't believe in miracles perhaps you've forgotten you are one.

— Jesse Joseph

OCCASIONALLY, WE WILL HAVE PATIENTS WHO DEFY THE ODDS. IF they have some unique quality of character that gives them an advantage over the other souls who populate our corridors, I have yet to discern it. Often, they are not who you expect. Through my years of witnessing courage, determination, and compassion, my mind inevitably drifts back to three who had many things in common, especially an insane commitment to a task. They were naturally optimistic and grateful. And, through all their suffering, they remained, at heart, children.

Sam had everything going for him: A loving and supportive wife, two children he adored, a great community, a positive attitude, and he was incredibly fit, a tae kwon do instructor and sixth-degree black belt in karate. He ran a martial arts school, ate clean, and meditated daily. Sam wasted little time in wondering why he developed leukemia, instead focusing on understanding his opponent and the treatments available. When I first met him, I was struck by his confidence and presence. Though sitting on a hospital bed, he was dressed not in the awkward gown we provide, but his own clothing. His eyes were steady and warm, his manner marked with respect for his medical team — proper, gracious, but not stuffy. He held himself with military poise.

When I introduced myself as the chaplain, Sam was keenly interested in understanding my role. It was exciting for him to find someone familiar with meditation, energy, and consciousness, as well as the part diet and exercise play in recovery. Our conversations were rich and deep, and I was honored that he came to see me as his cancer coach, just as he was a coach to so many in the skills of defense.

Sam was scheduled to receive a MUD transplant. His treatment began without incident, but we knew within three weeks he would hit some rough spots. Sure enough, on day fourteen post-transplant, mouth sores erupted and digestion ceased as his intestines purged themselves. By day twenty-one his liver and kidneys were failing, while his starving body ravaged muscle tone for protein. Sam withered from the model of fitness to a frail ghost of who he had been. During the spiral, we explored fear as both his opponent and his teacher. Every moment presented him with an opportunity to engage that force using the skill he had learned in martial arts: to understand your foe, to use the energy of attack against it, to remain centered and self-aware while opening to the flow of *qi*, the life force that, in Chinese culture, pervades all things.

Sam also explored his spirituality. Already a practicing Catholic, prayer was a daily part of life for him and his family. That connection moved to a much deeper level, through the stages of bargaining, petition, and rescue, to a connection of communing, of simply being in the presence of Spirit. This did not always go well. There was a period when Sam felt completely overwhelmed and trapped in fear. So, I introduced him to *Tonglen*, a Buddhist meditation in which he focused on the five other transplant patients in the rooms around his, drawing in the harsh reality of their experience which he knew too well, then sending compassion back into their bodies; breathing in their suffering, breathing out his light. By using his compassion for others he returned to his own sense of agency and choice. Sam also became more compassionate with his own suffering, which returned him to himself. *I understand* became his mantra. And in affirming that, Sam also affirmed his ability to be fully present to his own journey, to fully participate in his healing. Moving through this, he eventually found a deeper presence within himself, learned how to work with the shifting horizon of hope, compassionately forgiving and restoring his own heart to divine resonance.

Sam also did what he knew best: he trained. Even when his skeletal form could not rise from the bed, he trained. Leg lifts, crunches, arm raises. It began so slowly, one every few hours. It built incrementally, with his new target always 10 percent ahead of his previous one. Inching forward, eventually he was able to do a hundred crunches, and this before he was able to stand! When that victory was reached, Sam added squats while holding on to the foot of the bed. He started with one. The next day, two. The next, three. He charted all of this on the giant white board at the foot of his bed. He drank high protein, vitamin-rich smoothies until he could eat, which he then did in very small amounts. I'm convinced these cumulative steps, done with consistency and compassion, were as significant to his recovery as the treatments he received.

On leaving the hospital ten weeks after his transplant, Sam showed me a video of his last examination to achieve his sixth dan, or black belt level. It was poetry in motion to watch such power and agility. His goal now was to continue to the seventh dan, a dream that had been derailed by his diagnosis. He also planned to expand his school. Having witnessed his staggering commitment to healing while confined to four walls for over two months, I had no doubt Sam would achieve this dream.

THE SECOND REMARKABLE SURVIVOR WAS BOB. THIS QUIRKY AND ECCEN- tric young man was a mathematical and engineering prodigy, a musician, and a craftsman. Bob was also passionate about learning. Questions on the medical aspects of his care were ongoing but always asked from a desire to partner with the nurses and doctors, as well as to calm his ever-present mother. Diagnosed with lymphoblastic lymphoma, he considered all his options, while trusting the expertise of his medical team. Like Sam with his amplified attention to detail, Bob was able to focus on a goal and do everything he could to achieve it, yet he did this driven by his vision, not his anxiety. He was reaching for life, not running from his death. Bob's relaxed demeanor enabled him to roll with the side effects of treatment without too much attachment or need to control.

In his words, "I have little desire to compete, but a strong desire to win. So, if you have any chance, I say swing till your arms fall off. If not, then let it go."

This resulted in a remarkable endurance, especially as Bob developed acute pancreatitis due to a rare allergic reaction to the chemotherapy. He did have age in his favor; survival is good for younger patients with this disease, but it's not good if you can't tolerate the treatment. As we watched, his weight plummeted, his youthful body shrank to a skeletal form, and soon he was poised on the edge of consciousness. Even there, he would steadily, methodically inch toward health; a sip of water, a smile and joke, a humbling dedication to gratitude and his health goals. I was astonished when he walked into my office two years after treatment. His body was transformed. Bob had connected with a trainer, focusing on building muscular strength instead of mass, and he practiced meditation every day. He was better than before and credited cancer for the transformation. In addition, he started his own company doing custom guitar fabrication and inlay work, then moved his skill to fabricating bionic knee braces to enhance the strength and power of leg muscles.

DEBORAH WAS SO UNASSUMING. A DIMINUTIVE WOMAN, SHE HAD FROM THE start wanted to know nothing about her cancer or the treatment. Quiet and modest as a mouse, she'd just say, "Do what you gotta do." Her cancer was rare, very dangerous, and very difficult to treat. Deborah's sister donated the stem cells, but the engraftment didn't go smoothly. Now months had passed in the isolation room that protects patients from the germs we are unknowingly bathed in daily. To her it felt like a prison. Yet her pleasant, even temper didn't fail. She suffered mouth sores, diarrhea, rashes, weight loss, and profound weakness. She did not rise from the bed for over a month. We waited and waited for her counts to rise, for vitality to return. Like the others, she inched toward it. I was the only person she talked with about death, but it wasn't her own mortality that opened the discussion.

Deborah had worked as a personal care provider, mainly with senior citizens. She had witnessed many deaths, and some of them were marked by that amazing energy of spirit that fills the room. She did not, however, feel she would die, not this time round. What was the motivation that kept her going? Her grandkids. They were her greatest gift. They expanded her world and her heart in ways she could never have imagined. She had more love to give them, and she was determined to have the time to do it. It took half a year for health to return to the point when she could move from our hospital to one closer to her home, driven purely, it seemed, by love and determination. No passionate purpose, no profound faith, only her will and trusting her life still had a purpose.

THE SECRET INGREDIENTS

WHAT WAS IT ABOUT THESE INDIVIDUALS THAT ENABLED THEM TO NOT only survive but also thrive against all odds? They all possessed a quiet determination. They focused their inner resources to do the best they could. They did not believe in mind over matter, but neither did they comply blindly with medical advice. They also focused their love in the moment. This is, I suspect, a critical quality. Love became a compass, guiding them to their best selves. Yet, it was never done with great effort or striving. It flowed naturally, without effort; these patients were never even aware of it.

This is consistent with research on what we call "remarkable survivors." They all share some fairly specific qualities:
- They have a deep belief in the body's innate healing wisdom.
- They have a strong sense of self-sufficiency, competency, and control.

- They have a fulfilling and enjoyable life, beyond the crisis of cancer.
- They have at least one strong, supportive, and trusted relationship.
- They are comfortable with the expression of both positive and negative emotions.
- They find meaning in the cancer experience and accept the diagnosis but not the prognosis.
- They work in partnership with health professionals and participate in decisions related to their treatment and well-being.
- They regularly participate in activities and practices that reduce stress.
- They show flexibility and willingness to try new things and/or make changes when something is no longer working.
- They undergo a spiritual transformation, an awakening of their true values, which brings renewed authenticity to their relationships.[51]

A spiritual transformation. As grand as this sounds, it happens in the deep waters of consciousness, not on the surface level of ego. We're talking about that connection to the numinous again, a new awareness marked not by hallelujahs and praise, but by silence and contemplation.

Caryle Hirshberg and Marc Barasch explored this in their examination of belief as the main variable in remarkable recoveries.[52] A wonderful aspect of this research is that it shows the majority of people did not start off so enlightened and empowered. In fact, they were just as shocked and afraid as the next patient. But they chose to use their cancer experience to amplify life and accelerate their conscious development. Tied into this belief is the most wonderful and frustrating phenomenon known to medical science: the placebo effect. This may provide the key to understanding remarkable recoveries, and invites both healthcare professionals and patients to make them not so remarkable, but perfectly natural.

When given fake medication or treatment, a staggering percentage of patients experience remission of symptoms, even complete healing. Forty percent of headache sufferers, half of those struggling with colitis, and over half of those with ulcer pain experienced relief. Across illnesses — depression, Parkinson's, infertility, asthma, and even cancer — a large number of patients experience improvement from the placebo effect.[53] The variable appears to be something not so remarkable after all: heartfelt care. Patients fared better — much better — when they believed in the medicine *and* experienced their healthcare team genuinely caring: taking time to sit instead of stand, making eye contact, compassionately touching, accurately empathizing, and supportively encouraging. This partnership of compassion and belief is very powerful in activating the body's own healing potential, which includes the releasing of natural opioids (pain killers), inducing the relaxation response (a fundamental healing state) and supporting a cascade of healing processes. Chaplains provide this compassionate care, but do so still separate from the conversations and encounters a patient has with their doctor or nurse. And simply providing this quality of compassion is not enough to transform everyone into a remarkable survivor — many still die. What is it, then, about those who defy the odds? I would propose it is from a shift in one's foundation at the spiritual level. These elusive qualities of consciousness ripple out to affect the mental, emotional, and physical levels in ways medication can't.

Let's return briefly to the question of why we get cancer. Most doctors would agree there is something going on between the mind and body. The Centers for Disease Control and Prevention (CDC) even states, "Intensive and prolonged stress can lead to ... health problems later in life including alcoholism, depression, eating disorders, heart disease, cancer, and other chronic diseases."[54] Remarkable survivors do not, however, invest time and energy unraveling the cord that ties each stressor to the disease. Again, their question is not, Why did I get cancer, but, What am I going to do with it. And what they do is use cancer for the advancement of love, by releasing any unresolved pain through forgiveness.

Medicine does not yet have a prescription for this. Whatever role consciousness plays in the ability to endure far beyond prognosis will remain a mystery outside the realm of science. But that doesn't mean you have to wait to for any breakthroughs. You can take action now by listening to the burdens of your heart, the unresolved wounds of your life, and sending gratitude and forgiveness to them, for they are connected to the original injury, and remedy, for your disease.

Dr. Alastair Cunningham is the author of the Healing Journey Program, a multistep program for patients with advanced cancer, in which participants did more than change diet and lifestyle — they changed their consciousness. Releasing emotional pain, practicing meditation, and incorporating daily spiritual exercises designed to help them resonate more fully with their eternal selves, rather than their ego selves, enabled deeper healing than chemotherapy could touch. Dr. Cunningham observed a significant extension in quality and length of life for those who followed the program and, sometimes, unexpected remissions among his participants.[55]

Physicians tend to vastly underestimate patients when it comes to the mystery of death.[56] Basing their calculation on what can be measured, it's no wonder they are pleasantly surprised, again and again. The biology of belief is simply not a variable that fits neatly into the curriculum of Western medicine. It makes doctors scratch their heads, nurses smile with relief, and patients and families praise God. I, too, offer a prayer of thanks and then sit to ponder what is going on. But is it a miracle? Families are quite comfortable embracing that term. They pray for God to fix things, they look for the elixir that will cure, and sometimes they get it. But remarkable survivors don't go there. They develop a comfort with death, while focusing on life in this moment. They don't just change their minds about cancer; they change their lives. And their lives, as a result, feel quite different, marked by the ability to pause and be aware of the private, painful beauty of just being; the sound of leaves rustling in the wind, the taste of hot soup on a cold day, the touch of a child's hand in yours, all of it more than enough for a full life. Mortality is held with gratitude. Excruciating enlightenment.

MIRACLES CONTINUE TODAY

WHAT OF THOSE TIMES WHEN IT REALLY DOES SEEM MIRACULOUS INTERvention took place? Not just a remission or amazing response to treatment, but an all-out spiritual healing? Many have recalled the miracles of Jesus, exercising supernatural power to heal the sick, even raise the dead. One story I love as a model of healing is found in Mark 5:25–34. Jesus felt energy flow from him to heal a woman who had chronic menstrual bleeding. She reached out, and grazing her hand against the hem of his robe, was restored:

> Now there was a woman who had been suffering from hemorrhages for twelve years. She had endured much under many physicians, and had spent all that she had; and she was no better, but rather grew worse. She had heard about Jesus, and came up behind him in the crowd and touched his cloak, for she said, "If I but touch his clothes, I will be made well." Immediately her hemorrhage stopped; and she felt in her body that she was healed of her disease.

This story has stuck with me for many reasons, in part because she risked her life by touching a rabbi while she had a menstrual flow. That was a ritual taboo for which she could have been killed. Desperation and disease drew her to cross any social boundary in order to reach out and connect with the Holy before her. Yet there are times when we have no energy to reach out. Instead, the Holy reaches us.

I think of Doug, who was supposed to be dying. He had not only defied his doctor's prognosis, but also sailed through every treatment we had given him since his brush with death a year ago. That was when he lay in ICU, liver failing, heart erratic, his wife and family gathered for the vigil. Doug recalls being able to hear them at his side, talking anxiously with the nurse, while the machines monitoring his body pulsed softly at his side. But he could sense something else as well, and he knew from it that this was not the end.

Doug sat in my office, trying to describe it a year later. "It was so weird. There was this energy, this orb next to me. No one else could see it, but it was floating right there," he said, extending his arm. "I don't know what it was, but it was giving me strength. I knew I wasn't going to die. So I grabbed the rails of the bed and freaked them all out. I pulled myself up, sat right up, and told them, 'I'm not going to die!' I knew it wasn't my time."

Doug was a guy who didn't want to know a lot about his cancer, didn't exhibit an obsessive drive to master all he put his mind to. He was an unassuming, hard-working, self-effacing, regular guy. Life had thrown him a nasty divorce, a vicious cancer, and little fortune to bank on. He rolled with whatever came. As a result of the encounter with the orb of light, his spirituality was vibrant and open, though very private.

"I must be here for some purpose, that's the only thing I can think of. But beats me if I know what it is!"

Anita Moorjani has been working on that question ever since her miracle healing. Author of *Dying to be Me*, she had a profound near-death experience in 2006 during her battle with cancer. Disconnecting from her body, she shifted to an expansive state of clarity, understanding how we are so much more than we realize. Anita was able to sense the feelings of her family, yet from her new state of consciousness, this was experienced without the emotional burden that so often dominates a patient's heart. The spirit of her father guided her to the knowledge that her body would heal, if she chose to return. And her body was in rough shape: emaciated, riddled with lymphoma, lemon-sized tumors, open wounds, reliance on life support, failing organs. Yet, in five weeks, she was well enough to return home — an unexplainable rate of recovery. Anita relates that during her near-death experience, she was shown how choices in life contributed to cancer developing, especially with regard to how she did not love herself. From this she also learned the importance of living fearlessly, celebrating the unique gift of who she is as an expression of divine consciousness.

This is the universal human affliction: separation from love. The woman who suffered from hemorrhaging in the biblical story knew it well. In addition to her physical misery, she also endured her community's rejection due to the ritual laws of purity at the time. These prevented her from even entering the temple to practice her faith. She was a spiritual and communal outcast. So, as a result of her healing, she was not only physically restored, but reconnected with the gift of herself, her life, and her place in society. The story continues with Jesus performing a social miracle as well, for he dismissed the oppressive rules of his culture, and instead treated her as a whole person, worthy of respect and love:

> Immediately aware that power had gone forth from him, Jesus turned about in the crowd and said, "Who touched my clothes?" And his disciples said to him, "You see the crowd pressing in on you; how can you say, 'Who touched me?'" He looked all around to see who had done it. But the woman, knowing what had happened to her, came in fear and trembling, fell down before him, and told him the whole truth. He said to her, "Daughter, your faith has made you well; go in peace, and be healed of your disease."[57]

God's healing is never one-dimensional. As such, it is never enough to ask for physical healing from God without addressing the other broken aspects of life. There is an assignment of love still to be done. This is, ultimately, the plan for each of us: we are to become love itself. That is the ultimate miracle, and it can come even if you die. Sometimes, that is the only way for it to happen. But we don't want that outcome. We pray, we plead, and we petition the powers that be to spare us that fate. What was that quality of consciousness that enabled her restoration? Jesus named it: faith. Perhaps our issue is not that we have it, but that we don't understand it. Faith is a state of connected consciousness. You experience God as immanent and transcendent, both flowing through you and infinitely greater than you, sustaining you in every moment. Far from being the conductor of your life, you are, instead, an instrument in a vast symphony being expressed from God.[58] Healing may then be understood as coming into tune with the sacred song.

PART 3

Consciousness:
The Journey Is Transformative

CHAPTER 11

THIRD TUMOR

Can you allow yourself to be impaled on the present moment?
— T. SCOTT McLEOD, *ALL THAT IS UNSPOKEN*

WE HAD MOVED FROM SASKATCHEWAN TO MY SECOND PARISH IN Halifax, Nova Scotia. The opportunity enabled us to be closer to my family, experience the ocean again, and opened opportunities for my wife to attend any of three universities in the city. Settling in also meant securing a good family physician. Fortunately, an excellent one practiced just down the hill from our new home. Unfortunately, she was not taking new patients. Dr. G. was among the most recommended family docs in the city. Patients raved about her insight, warmth, and professional ability. Determined to meet her and discuss our care needs, I walked into her clinic and asked for an appointment.

The receptionist was friendly but firm. "I'm sorry, Dr. G is not accepting new patients at this time."

"I understand," I said, as I took a pen from the desk and wrote one word on a sticky note: pheochromocytoma. "Please give this to her." Perhaps it was the boldness of the move; more likely, I was simply lucky. The receptionist disappeared with the note, and a moment later emerged with an intrigued physician.

"On one condition," Dr. G. said with a smile, "I get to see you in the hospital." Simple enough.

"Agreed," I replied.

We then formally introduced ourselves and began what would be a wonderful relationship of medical care, emotional support, and mutual appreciation that continues to this day, over twenty years later. A family physician is your first line of care, and I am deeply grateful for Dr. G.'s expertise and support through the years. Her knowledge of this rare condition has been invaluable, and through her we were able to find an excellent endocrinologist. Together, we discussed the difficulty of distinguishing between early cancer symptoms and normal signs of stress and anxiety, and developed a plan for early detection. That plan paid off: within four years of the previous surgery, the catecholamines began to rise again.

An MIBG scan uses a radioactive tracer to light up neuroendocrine tumors. My previous ones had been in the bladder and femoral artery. I prayed this third one would be in the same area, not on my adrenal glands. That would require removing them and using hormone therapy for the rest of my life. The tumor could also be in my heart or brain, resulting in an even more dangerous operation. However, the results came back blank — nothing lit up. While metabolically active, the tumor was too small to appear on the scan. We would have to let it grow. This meant I would get reacquainted with my symptoms: fingernails turning light blue from constricting capillaries, a cold sweat and dizziness whenever I became anxious, massive stomach cramps and diarrhea. I'm fine, I'm fine, would be my mantra as I paced and breathed into my twisting gut. The body never lies, but the mind will be the first to deceive you. So, try as I might to block the anxiety, I could not block the truth of my cold hands and ghostly pallor.

Waiting is always the hardest. You wait for a test. You wait for a procedure. You wait for anything to happen because until it does, the cancer is growing. You imagine it in your body; you know it's getting worse, and you want it out. It was always on my mind, and I found myself blurting out statements that betrayed the civilized façade.

One well-intentioned neighbor asked how I was, and to my astonishment and hers, I coldly replied, "I have cancer, how the hell do you think I am?" Regret filled me before the sentence was finished. Suddenly, waiting for the tumor to explode and end my life didn't seem reason enough to be uncivil. I was withdrawn and sullen with my family, and apathetic at work in my parish. I could never forget the warning from the doctor when the previous tumor was identified: this is pheochromocytoma — to feel can be fatal. But emotionally flatlining only made things worse. I become brooding and detached. In my heart I entertained the secret world of death while chatting at the supper table, playing with my son, smiling with the neighbors. My self-talk was filled with bravado: I'm afraid, but won't allow it to come close. It could kill me. But hey, I'm a veteran of this by now. I'll sail through, as I always do. What pretense! Those who cared for me weren't fooled for a minute, but they graciously allowed my denial while witnessing my slow implosion.

If there was anything constructive I gained from this experience, it was to learn meditation as a survival tool. Many think of meditation as tuning out, quieting the mind, but it's quite the opposite. To meditate is to fully show up with what is here and now, to tune in to the whole mess. Through compassionate presence, you change your relationship to that mess. As much as I needed to calm down, reaching for that goal only sabotaged the attempt. By trying to fix myself, I suppressed the reality of my own experience. And whatever you suppress within, you give power to. My real goal, then, was not to get it together, but to get real. Be authentic. Be present. Move into this crisis with full awareness. It was terrifying. As I inched toward the fear, my fingers would turn cold and numb. Cramps wrung out my bowels, and the pulse of blood loaded with adrenaline throbbed against the skin of my neck. So, I orbited the edge of anxiety. I mentally danced around reality. Watching myself do that was enough at first.

The benefits of meditation have been well documented. In particular, it influences the relaxation response and supports psychological well-being,[59] thus greatly reducing mortality in adults with heart disease.[60] That was my target, since pheochromocytoma produces an excess of noradrenaline — precisely the chemical that triggers heart attacks. As a Lutheran pastor, I actually had little training in meditation, or even prayer, for that matter. Ours was a heavy academic program, focused on theology, parish administration, liturgy, and counseling. Ironically, in a way, my tumors opened me to a deeper connection with God and myself far more than seminary training ever did.

Mindfulness is a similar practice to meditation, but instead of using a mantra or deep contemplative practice, mindfulness is a way of being. It is conscious living. This includes mindful eating (food tastes so much better!), mindful relationships (noticing how I extend or withhold love), mindful speech (words are events, after all),[61] and physical awareness. This last one was interesting. I would take only a moment to scan my body, using it as the barometer of being, one that would not deceive me as easily as my mind did. I noticed where and how I was holding tension, adjusted my posture, and remembered to smile. Three options would then present themselves: I could do nothing, I could criticize my own thoughts and feelings, or I could practice compassion for myself and gently move toward conscious health.

Many Christians feel uncomfortable with meditation, associating it with Eastern spiritual traditions. However, there is a strong tradition of it within Christianity, called "centering prayer." This is a silent communing with the Spirit, being still and knowing God (or rather, embracing vulnerability and being known). Rather than talking to God or making a petition, this form of prayer is more like feeling the company of the Divine. One can use a mantra, such as *maranatha*, which means both "Come, Lord!" and "Our Lord has come!" Notice the exclamation — there's a lot of energy in this word! It expresses the desire for the divine Spirit to come to your heart, as well as the affirmation that it has already happened. I loved this dual meaning, for it met both my need for God's presence and knowing that God was already within me.

Come, Lord. Come. It was the only phrase that brought me compassionately to my pain. It was the only phrase that broke open my tears and safely released the pressure of imagined outcomes. And it was only possible when I was alone, when it felt safe to cry. As a wise patient pointed out, we wear emotional armor not to protect ourselves from what comes at us from others, but to contain what lies within. Eventually, the armor corrodes, gaps appear, and we discover we didn't need it after all. This does not happen all at once! There were plenty of times when I took off my armor, then put it on again whenever someone asked that common question: How are you?

This experience showed me how we spend so much mental energy avoiding ourselves, and that the greatest tragedy in such an escape is we cannot, then, encounter the presence of God (who is found only in the present moment). Every Sunday service I led that year became an opportunity for me to not only believe in God but also to believe *into* God. They were invitations for me to open to the divine Spirit and drill deep into peace, quieting my autonomic nervous system, overriding the fight-or-flight mechanism through compassionate presence and the prayerful desire to merge my consciousness with the Divine. This is difficult to describe, a floating feeling, both heavy and light, a prayer of longing to disappear: Maranatha, maranatha. Come to me, Lord. I am reaching through my mortality to your eternity, where the light is infused with love. I am aching for you. I am held. I am home.

Some days I did that well, others not so much. But what a profound opportunity to deepen one's faith! At the time, I couldn't imagine how this would also train me in supporting others as they left this world through cancer, or lost loved ones to it.

The surgery I ultimately required went well. The recovery did not. An infection spread rapidly after I was discharged. Weakness, fever, and delirium were complicated by my stupidity and stubbornness to stay in the comfort of home. Finally, with a temperature peaking at 104°F, I relinquished the illusion of control, and shivered with rigors in the safety of a hospital bed.

Late that night I struggled to sleep, restless and tossing. Feeling a presence in the room, I turned to see a figure in the dark silhouetted against the curtain drawn about the bed. I thought it must be the nurse and called out. Suddenly she disappeared. I lay bewildered by peace, suddenly still and heavy, and slumbered until morning.

It was early when my own nurse came to check my temperature, clearly surprised when he found me sitting up and reading in the pre-dawn light.

"Good morning!" I said with a smile.

"Well, this is good to see," he said. "Feeling better? You were having quite the night."

"Yes, don't recall much of it, except that other nurse who came in to check on me."

"Who?" he asked. "I was the only one caring for you. No one's been in here but me."

CHAPTER 12

YOUR ENERGETIC ANATOMY

Why should not the proximity of the human body … exert upon
a neighboring human body, by means of an aura or radiation, an
influence which stimulates or tranquilizes the other's nerves?

— KARL VON REICHENBACH, 1844

ENERGY FLOWED FROM JESUS IN THE STORY FROM MATTHEW, AND AS part of the ministry he commissioned to his disciples, he instructed them to lay their hands on the sick as well, healing in his name.[62] While I took this seriously, in my training as a minister we never explored it beyond the stories themselves. There was an unspoken agreement that miracles were part of the past, the folklore of faith not to be expected from amateurs such as us. At best, we were inadequate conduits of such grace. And yet, there always seemed to be more at hand.

Healing is part of most faith traditions; accounts are hardly limited to Christianity. If there was a quality of consciousness that activated or released this energetic equilibrium, I was sure it must be a universal human potential. Then I stumbled across one of many secular expressions of the phenomena. It was called "Therapeutic Touch." Here was a practice built on what I had learned of the laying-on-of-hands in seminary, but explored from a completely new angle, a clinical application of a spiritual phenomenon designed for use in hospitals.

Ironically, though it's called Therapeutic Touch, no touch is actually required, as the practice was developed for use even if a hospital patient had an infection or was in isolation. The process is deceptively simple and, to be honest, it looks a bit odd. Practitioners mindfully center themselves, focusing on the present moment and directing or tuning their own consciousness to a state of balance and awareness. This is done, as with all meditative practices, simply through the power of intention, awareness, and the breath. For myself, I focus upon a compassionate heart and invite God to flow through me. (While Therapeutic Touch is independent of religious tradition and belief, it is still a spiritual practice, and partnering with the Divine is how I experience it.) The effectiveness of the treatment depends mostly upon my being able to "plug in" while also getting out of my own way.

The treatment begins with my hands passing over the person's body, quickly assessing and sensing any imbalance in their energy field. The patient may be awake or asleep, it does not matter. I work with the field, clearing and balancing it through what appear to be brushing gestures. All this is happening about three to six inches above the patient, though sometimes I go much higher. I check my work with another scan, and then lightly touch the patient's feet to ground the energy and help it flow through the body. Grounding may be done several times throughout the treatment, and some practitioners touch more often. Patients are surprised and deeply moved by the profound peace that comes upon them. This is such a welcome shift from the continual worry and struggle of cancer.

Studies, though still small, are expanding our understanding of the interplay between consciousness and biology. While Therapeutic Touch is among the most researched of energy healing modalities, many of the studies have not met the rigorous standards of academic publication. Of course, there are several reasons why this is simply not practical: studies of that size are expensive; paranormal phenomena tend not to lend themselves to replication but are one-time events; and it is difficult, if not impossible, to account for the variability of consciousness itself, especially when we don't have a clue as to what it really is! There is excellent work being done, nonetheless, much of which can be found in a wonderful tome, *Irreducible Mind: Toward a Psychology for the 21st Century*. Bridging cognitive psychology, neuroscience, and parapsychology, the point is driven home, example after example: mind is independent of the brain, and it continues after death.[63]

Among the very good studies on Therapeutic Touch is one that examined the effect of healing energy on bone cancer. The cancerous bone cells sat in dishes alongside healthy tissue. Therapeutic Touch was performed twice a week for ten minutes. The samples that received treatments had a significant increase in healthy cell growth for the normal tissue, while the cancer cells died more rapidly. By examining the effect on cells in isolation, the researchers removed many of the variables that emerge with a human subject.[64]

Another study found great improvement in the well-being of twenty subjects with terminal cancer after only three treatments.[65] Indeed, hundreds of research studies have shown similar results. The success I have achieved with patients has left me grateful for a modality that complements and brings an intelligent theory of healing to my religious practice. However, as much as it can be a valuable method of connecting to wonder, hope, and peace, for some it can actually be terrifying.

A Silvery Light

WHILE I HAD USED THERAPEUTIC TOUCH IN MY PARISH AFTER SERVICES, along with workshops exploring the nature of spirit, energy, and healing, in the hospital I was more hesitant. Even though I was a chaplain, and moving my hands over someone while silently centering in the Spirit was actually within my scope of practice, I brought Therapeutic Touch slowly and carefully into the cancer program over several years. Treatments would be given for nausea, pain management, and anxiety. Gradually patients were telling the nurses how much better it made them feel, and then, one day, a nurse asked me for a treatment for herself.

Pam had sprained her ankle some weeks back, and on this day it was throbbing in the heat. She requested a treatment, so I rolled my chair up to hers at the nursing desk. I was unaware of Michelle, our charge nurse, standing nearby, watching as I assessed the field about Pam's leg. It was only a minute or two into the treatment when Michelle exclaimed in shock and fear at what she saw: a smoky apparition snaked around my fingers and made her catch her breath and question her sanity. It was the energy field.

Unable to avert her eyes, she stammered, "What are you doing to me?!"

"I'm not doing anything to you, Michelle. I'm treating Pam." While Pam was comfortable with occasionally seeing energy fields and quite familiar with Therapeutic Touch, Michelle had come from a different school. Rigorous science, material reality, what you see is what you get had been her world up to this point. As she looked down at my hands moving about Pam's leg, what she saw was surreal: a silvery fluid light flowing between us, responding to the pull of my fingers and delicate proximity of my palms.

"But I can see it, I can see stuff around her ankle, I can see … stop it. Stop it! You're freaking me out!"

"Relax," I replied. "It's just the energy field, and you're seeing it because you can, not because of me."

Pam's confirmation did nothing to calm Michelle. "Oh, yeah, and I can feel it, too. My skin's tingling, feels like Dave's pulling the pain right out with his fingers. You should try it sometime."

That was enough to drive Michelle over the edge, and she pulled away from the two of us, shaking her head. Finishing the treatment, I calmly explained to Michelle that while we all have a physical body, we also have an energetic anatomy, two aspects of what it is to be human and alive. I informed her that Therapeutic Touch originated as a nursing practice, based on ancient wisdom of the body's energy field as well as good science. But she was still upset.

"My life and my career have always been based on hard science, what you can see and touch. That was nothing I've ever seen before."

"Well," I offered, "maybe you actually have the gift of being able to see the field. It's certainly not something I did to you. All you did was look, and it was there."

Pam's ankle felt much better after the treatment; however, Michelle did not. It took her several months to come to terms with what she saw. Her worldview had completely changed, and understandably, that takes time to adapt to. Notions of health, illness, treatment … all were challenged, and the implications for her practice as a nurse — and as a human being — would take years to realize. How much more so for our culture.

LUMINESCENT BEINGS

ARE YOU MORE THAN YOUR BODY? ARE YOU ACTUALLY A SPIRITUAL BEING having a physical experience? And if so, how can you tap into that level of consciousness to reverse cancer and transform your life? In this chapter and following, we will explore how, exactly, we are more than flesh and blood, and the connection between thought and matter that makes healing from the spiritual level possible.

Skepticism and ridicule are common responses, scoffing at the notion that the energy field exists at all. These arise both from incredulity, as Michelle experienced, and from a lack of awareness of advancements in technologies that have enabled scientists to observe the biofield, as well as see the interactions of healers. Yet, even compared to a sensitive photomultiplier, which detects light particles emanating from a person's skin, the best instrument to detect the field continues to be another human being.

This may have been the case throughout history, as artists and authors have depicted halos about the heads of holy figures and heroes in all cultures. Plato described the light emanating from warriors. Buddhist and Hindu images show light radiating from the entire body in a flame-like dance. Even Egyptian images dating back three thousand years show similar radiance about the head and shoulders. This is not, of course, limited to ancient times or to mystics and psychics; the average person can see it too, just as Michelle could. And the aura emanates from everyone, not just the saints and exceptional ones among us. Without some awareness of the phenomena, though, the ability to sense this life force is often suppressed out of fear or dismissed as imagination, lost for the rest of a person's life.

It's not difficult to understand why. Those who claim the sight are often perceived as quacks, flighty and far beyond the fringe. One such person fits that description perfectly, a grandmotherly grinning figure who retained the ability from childhood through her ninety-five years. Dora Kunz was a prominent figure in the Theosophical Society of New York, and she claimed to see signs of imbalance and disease in people's auras. To test this, she collaborated in the 1930s with an immunologist, Dr. Otelia Bengtsson. He was studying patients with allergic conditions that were difficult to treat. Kunz observed what she believed to be emotional patterns within their auras and developed theories concerning their relationship to disease.[66]

While eccentric in her beliefs, her abilities and theories contributed much to the emerging field of energy medicine. It would occupy her whole life, and connect her, forty years later, with Dolores Krieger, a professor of nursing at New York University, who was also studying the healing effect of laying-on-of-hands. Together, they explored the abilities of several healers and developed a clinical application of the principles observed. They called it Therapeutic Touch. Krieger states, "In the final analysis, it is the healee (client) who heals himself. The healer or therapist, in this view, acts as a human energy support system until the healee's own immunological system is robust enough to take over."[67]

Therapeutic Touch is now taught at over 70 universities in North America and in over 100 countries, with over 1,000 studies and articles to date. It is part of a family of energy healing modalities, including qigong and reiki, shiatsu, pranic healing and acupuncture, among others. Many of these draw from ancient spiritual practices, but this new expression offered a more grounded explanation of the phenomena of healing.

The idea that we are luminescent beings is not unique. For thousands of years, philosophical and spiritual traditions have taught that the universe is composed of interacting matrices of energy derived from an intelligent and coherent source. In this worldview, there is an underlying unity to all consciousness, of which an individual is a localized expression.

Many Native American cultures view the individual as a system of energy comprised of physical, emotional, and spiritual components. Organs are understood to have their own characteristic rhythm and resonance within the greater body system. Sickness is a loss of resonance within the body, as well as within the community. Re-patterning through music, drumming, and chanting is instrumental in their methods of healing.

In the traditions of India, this energizing life force is "prana," permeating the environment and underlying the diversity of life. Prana responds to an individual's thoughts and emotions, which in turn impacts physical health. Biography becomes biology. This connection between thoughts, feelings, and the body has been understood to be self-evident for thousands of years.

In Chinese culture, the term is "qi" (or chi), an energy that supports life and tends toward higher states of order. This life principle is constantly flowing and characteristic to each individual. In health, there is balance and harmony. When qi becomes disordered, illness may result. The flow is organized in the human system through pathways or meridians. An acupuncturist can use small needles or pressure to regulate the flow of qi. As each meridian has an energetic link to a specific organ, acupuncture is an example of treating the physical form through the energetic field. According to the National Institutes of Health, acupuncture has been found to be effective in the management of chemotherapy-associated nausea and vomiting, controlling pain associated with surgery,[68] and relieving both acute and chronic pain.[69]

During Kunz's life, such ideas were foreign to Western medicine. Yet interesting things were emerging. While she was working with Bengtsson on healing and energy in the 1930s, on the other side of the world, Georges Lakhovsky, a Russian engineer, was thinking about the same thing. In 1925 he theorized that every living creature radiates energy, and that a cell's nucleus acts as an electrical oscillating circuit, similar to a radio transmitter. He developed the Multiple Wave Oscillator, which treated the body with healing frequencies, especially for those afflicted with cancer.[70] Interestingly, Dr. Disraeli Kobak, pioneer of ultrasound in medicine, invited Lakhovsky to New York University to continue his research in energy waves and healing. One cannot help but wonder if Kunz and Lakhovsky ever coordinated their work on the human energy field.

In 1910 biologist Alexander Gurwitsch developed the concept of morphogenetic fields. His theory proposes there is a higher matrix of signals, external to individual cells, which govern biological development. This meant that a cell was not controlled solely by its genetic contents, its chromosomes, but by its energetic environment.

Gurwitsch explored how these hidden signals could affect living tissue by placing onion plants in adjacent pots and adding a toxin to the soil of one. The other onions' root systems were fine when in adjacent quartz glass pots, but not if they were in silicon ones. Silicon filters ultraviolet light, so he concluded the plants communicated with each other through UV rays.[71]

Dr. Fritz-Albert Popp, a theoretical physicist at the University of Marburg, Germany, and founder of the International Institute of Biophysics, picked up morphogenic field theory in 1970. His groundbreaking work in biophotonics and quantum biology is explored through eight books and over fifty research papers. Popp discovered that benzo[a]pyrene, a cancer-inducing molecule, absorbed UV light and then emitted it at a new frequency. It was a light scrambler. He expanded his research to thirty-seven other chemicals. After controlled studies, he was able to predict which chemical would be carcinogenic by their absorption of UV light, which was then emitted at a different frequency. What he could not discover was the precise frequency (or frequencies) that would reverse the process, initiating healing within the body.

Though the early 1900s was an era of profound discovery, the work of Lakhovsky, Gurwitsch, and others remained esoteric. Then came Einstein's theory of special relativity, which showed that light and matter are just aspects of the same thing (simply put, matter is frozen light, and light is matter on the move). This was central in building a unified theory of reality, of explaining how all things are interrelated. Still, there was no room for consciousness in Einstein's equations. The idea of an energy field emanating from a body remained an oddity at best, and our ability to affect it through the power of the mind was relegated to the scope of psychics and religious mysticism. Advocates of the concept remained small voices in the academic community, but voices filled with enthusiasm and wonder, nonetheless.

Among those pioneers was another notable figure in science: Dr. Harold Saxton Burr, professor of anatomy at Yale School of Medicine. In his book *Blueprint for Immortality*, he explored what he called L-fields, or life fields. "The Universe," he wrote, "in which we find ourselves and from which we cannot be separated is a place of Law and Order. It is not an accident, nor chaos. It is organized and maintained by an electro-dynamic field capable of determining the position and movement of all charged particles. For nearly half a century, the logical consequences of this theory have been subjected to rigorously controlled conditions and met with no contradictions."[72] Here, finally, was convincing understanding of the underlying cause of disease from a leading figure in the health sciences: illness was the result of subtle changes in bioelectric fields caused by dissonance with fields in the local environment.

Others voices joined in. Dr. W. Ross Adey, researcher with the American Institute of Stress, studied the psychophysiological effects of weak magnetic fields and communication between cells. His research explored how cells "whisper" together through their membranes, which vibrate in their own particular electromagnetic communities. Adey found that if communication between cells is compromised or stops, they do something remarkable and frightening. They begin to clone, meaning they become cancerous. Cancer is cells growing out of control, unregulated and in opposition to their biological community.

People, too, much like the cell, are naturally driven to find in community another soul who mirrors them but is not a clone. Simply put, we seek friendship. When this is not established at an early age, narcissism may result, an attempt to mirror the self. When we are physically isolated we may even begin to talk to ourselves. If we are emotionally isolated, we may produce multiple personalities — if the self cannot find community, it will invent it. From birth, our emotional system searches for resonating contact, not duplicating or identical sameness. Community and diversity are as essential to the health of humanity as they are to the health of our microscopic components. One can equally expand that truth to encompass all of reality.

The view that humans and the environment are inseparable from the universe is a fundamental component of modern physics. Victor Guillemin, in discussing quantum field theory, states, "fields alone are real, they are the substance of the universe."[73] And in a classic paper first published in 1935 — the same period in which Kunz's work was developing — Burr and Northrop affirmed in their essay "The Electro-Dynamic Theory of Life," that "the pattern and organization of any biological system is established by a complex electrodynamic field."[74]

Health, then, is a term for balance, harmony, or healthy relationship on all levels. Beyond your skin, it is with the environment, your community, your family. Within yourself, it continues among biological systems (nervous, skeletal, digestive, etc.), between individual cells, within them, to the atomic and subatomic levels, and beyond. At the most basic level is the energy of consciousness (which we will explore in chapter 13). And this is where "you" come in, so to speak. Your consciousness, your mind, can cause a shift in the field to support health through releasing thought patterns and feelings which have, to this point, perpetuated separation, pain, and suffering. The ripple effect through your body is tied to the restoration of your relationships, your past, and your identity as a being who has, fundamentally, never been separated from God. This is the identity and truth, I believe, that Jesus maintained. As for us, well, we stumble awkwardly along, oblivious of the energetic nature of reality around us, believing the incessant illusion.[75]

While it has long been known that activities of cells and tissues generate electrical fields that can be detected on the skin's surface, the laws of physics demand that any electrical current generate a corresponding magnetic field in the surrounding space. Since these fields were too tiny to detect, biologists assumed they could have no significance on the body. This picture began to change in 1963, when Gerhard Baule and Richard McFee of the Department of Electrical Engineering, Syracuse University, detected the biomagnetic field projected from the human heart. In 1970 David

Cohen of the Massachusetts Institute of Technology (MIT) confirmed the heart measurements, using a SQUID magnetometer (Superconducting Quantum Interference Device). By 1972 Cohen had improved the sensitivity of his instrument, enabling him to measure magnetic fields around the head produced by brain activities.[76]

Subsequently, it has been discovered that all tissues and organs produce specific magnetic pulsations, which have come to be known as biomagnetic fields. These are likely the morphogenetic fields Gurwitsch postulated in the early 1900s. Interestingly for energy healers, only the magnetic pulsations of the brain and the hands share the same resonance. Photomultipliers can also detect the human energy field by measuring light particles emerging from the hands and foreheads of the healers. That field is strongest at the heart, and when one achieves a harmonious link between the brain and the heart, this field leaps out from the individual to affect the local environment.[77]

Others have confirmed these findings. Orthopedic surgeon Robert Becker developed a device that mapped out the electrical resistance on the body, and it corresponds directly with the Chinese map of the energetic anatomy, complete down to each meridian line and acupuncture point. Becker and others confirmed what had been known for thousands of years: this energy field alters in shape and strength with physiological and psychological changes. It responds to the environment and to other people's energy fields. Every aspect of who and what we are is reflected in the field.[78] And, if that doesn't make you feel vulnerable enough, we are naked to those who may, intuitively and astonishingly, be able to sense the field. That was Michelle's surprise when she saw me treating Pam's ankle, and it shook the foundation of her world. No wonder there is so much resistance in medicine to incorporating this in the standard curriculum.

Ironically, energy medicine has been there all along and is found in a first-year medical textbook. Biochemist Albert Lehninger, author of the standard reference *Principles of Biochemistry*, which has been used in medical schools since 2000, explains that cellular processes throughout the body happen almost simultaneously, not through chemicals or hormones but via biophotons. Low-level light emissions turn out to be a common property of all living cells, with up to one hundred photons of light emitted every second for every square centimeter of area. That's very, very faint, yet it takes the absorption of only a single photon to close one thousand or more ion channels and change the cell membrane's electric potential.[79] This ability of cells to communicate with light is now being explored through the field of optogenetics, in which biological processes are controlled and manipulated through the introduction of photosensitive proteins that react to light shining both inside and, surprisingly, outside the body.[80] Sound familiar? Reichenbach, Lakhovsky, Gurwitsch, Becker … scientists ridiculed in their day are applauding from the grave.

Compassionate presence turns out to be so much more than kindness; it is the active engagement of your own bioenergetic field, one that is infused with wisdom and power to assist another person in restoring health and vitality. The strongest field, interestingly, comes from the heart. The Institute of HeartMath has done extensive work in this area, demonstrating that the heart's electromagnetic field can be five thousand times stronger than that produced by the brain. It can be measured several feet away from the body, but may be global in its reach, if understood as a psychic phenomenon.[81]

Dr. Margaret Moga, associate professor of anatomy and cell biology at Indiana University School of Medicine, conducted her own experiments that verified shifts in the 8–10 Hz range of the magnetic field emitted by practitioners performing healing treatment.[82] These studies suggest the frequencies Dr. Fritz-Albert Popp was looking for in understanding the role UV light plays in the health of the body reside in the 8–10 Hz band. Interestingly, this is also the dominant resonance of the magnetic field of the planet.

All disease, indeed all metabolic processes, first starts at the level of subtle energy. Before any chemical reaction can occur, at least one electron must be activated by a photon with a certain wavelength and enough energy. Therapeutic Touch operates on this principle, with the practitioner as the instrument mapping out the magneto-electric balance of the body and modulating energy through the quality of the practitioner's own consciousness to initiate resonance and achieve balance.

A Massage of Light

I recall one therapeutic touch session in which the patient not only experienced the energy but also accurately described the photonic emissions. What made this treatment particularly wonderful is that it was not initiated by the patient or nurse, but by the doctor who caught me walking by the nursing desk. She was in a huddle with two nurses and a pharmacist.

"David! Get over here." A curious greeting. "Listen, we've got a patient in room 92 who's having a hell of a time with nausea and vomiting. The chemo we're about to give him will send him over the edge, but he's allergic to the antiemetics. Only thing that works for him is marijuana, and we can't give him that here."

Antiemetics are drugs that block the chemicals that cause nausea. There are many to choose from. If he was allergic to all of them, he must be quite sensitive.

"You do that magic thing with your hands to help patients. Think it would work on him?"

"Sure," I said, "can give it a try. But it's not magic, it's a clinical application of modulating …"

"Whatever!" she interrupted. "Just go do that thing you do." I was thrilled, for it showed me how Therapeutic Touch, that "weird hand-waving voodoo" I do, was being accepted by staff and physicians. Walking to the room with the nurse, I had only one thought: I hope this works! The patient was lying on the bed, a fellow in his forties, relaxed and friendly.

"Hey, I'm Dave, the chaplain. I hear the stuff we usually give for nausea doesn't work too well with you, and wanted to offer an alternative."

"Man, that'd be great!" he replied. "I just can't take the meds, really messes me up, can't breathe, I get this rash. What've you got?"

"Well, it's not a drug, it's kind of a relaxation tool called Therapeutic Touch. Basically, I move my hands over your body, head to toe, working with your energy field to balance and clear it while the chemo goes in. Might sound weird, but we use it a lot around here for nausea, and the team thought it might help, especially in your case."

He seemed willing to try anything. "Sounds cool. What do I have to do?" "Well, nothing, really. Just lie back. Shouldn't take longer than ten minutes. If it works, it's because I plugged in, so to speak. It all depends on me." This instruction and reassurance takes the pressure off the patient, who often feels overwhelmed and powerless. The effectiveness really does depend on my ability to deeply center myself, opening my heart chakra through compassion, and modulating my own field through intent, just as the HeartMath studies explore.

The patient happily reclined as the nurse prepared the chemotherapy infusion. I began the treatment by centering, modulating awareness with the breath, and then gently passing my hands over the patient to quickly assess the field.

The treatment continued for ten minutes, the duration of the chemo infusion. I focused on being compassionately present. During a treatment it is the patient who leads; my task is to "listen with my skin"; I have tingling sensations, feel changes in temperature and even what feels like air density. It's all quite intuitive as I try to respond to what his field presents.

While I did this, the nurse focused on his heart rate and blood pressure, checking his skin and breathing for any adverse reaction. None. He seemed sound asleep. As the saline ran, I sat by his bed with the nurse, who had a tray ready should he have any sign of nausea. Then we noticed him stir.

"How ya doing?" I quietly asked. He stretched, yawned, smiled.

"Oh, man, that was nice, I don't remember the last time I felt so relaxed. I could feel your hands moving over me. It was like a massage of light." The nurse was smiling, so relieved he hadn't reacted adversely to the chemo. I smiled, too, feeling profound gratitude for being part of this beautiful, mysterious process.

"So happy to hear that. Just rest in that for a while. I'll check on you later." It's important for a person not to rise immediately after a healing session, as the energy is still at work throughout the body, and one can compromise its lasting effect by shifting out of that relaxed state too soon.

Back at the nursing desk, the doctor sat charting another patient. "How'd it go?" she asked, without looking up.

"Great," I said. "He had no reaction to the chemo, moved nicely into the relaxation response, and is resting comfortably."

"Good job," she responded, and then moved on to her next patient, while I made note on the session. What does one write in a medical chart after waving their hands above a person to counter a biochemical process that should have left him retching for hours? "Patient was given Therapeutic Touch on referral from medical team for prevention of nausea and vomiting. Patient is allergic to antiemetics. Responded well, entering relaxation response within one minute, and remained relaxed throughout chemo infusion. Will follow." That last note was important. Nausea may not begin until hours after the chemo is given. Fortunately, he remained comfortable throughout the day, and was able tolerate the treatment he needed, thanks to some unconventional care.

This is just a sample of the growing body of knowledge reshaping our understanding of what it means to be human, to be so much more than flesh and bone. The implications are staggering. Bioenergetics tells us that we do not stop at our skin, that there is no such thing as a private thought, that intention is direction in effecting change in our lives and in the world. But does it point to more? Could it be a window to understanding the spiritual world? To tackle that, we have to consider what consciousness is.

CHAPTER 13

THE CONSCIOUSNESS CONUNDRUM

*About all we know of consciousness is that it has something
to do with the head, rather than the foot.*

— NICK HERBERT, PHYSICIST

ARE YOU HERE? SEEMS LIKE A RIDICULOUS QUESTION, YET IT IS THE bedrock of scientific inquiry on the most perplexing problem of all, that of consciousness. We all experience it: you're reading this book, aware of my words, your thoughts, and your body in your environment. How could this be questioned, and why does it matter? Because the dominant opinion in the scientific world is that the "you" you think you are doesn't exist.

Thomas S. Kuhn, author of the classic 1962 study *The Structure of Scientific Revolutions*, explains that the process of a paradigm shift begins when a persistent anomaly is observed with increasing frequency. When alternate theories are proposed that break the pattern of established perspectives, proponents are ridiculed, dismissed, rejected. Pioneers always act against considerable risk. Gradually, the view is tolerated until someone makes a breakthrough, which sweeps the new paradigm to center stage.

(Often it takes one generation to pass away before the next can move forward with the new paradigm.)

Kuhn writes: "A scientific revolution is a noncumulative developmental episode in which an older paradigm is replaced in whole or in part by an incompatible new one ... the normal scientific tradition that emerges from a scientific revolution is not one incompatible but often actually incommensurable with that which has gone before." This means the new model cannot be measured or qualified by the old. However, the new model integrates the dynamics of previous paradigms. This is exactly the case in the study of consciousness; the most transformative topic that will revolutionize our species once science embraces it. Unfortunately, that is not going to happen without a lot of heat, for those who propose that consciousness is the fundamental reality from which ours arises are treated as Galileo was by the church in his day, when he proposed the Earth is not the center of the universe: They are condemned. They are heretics. They are thrown out of the club. Which is odd, considering that radical perspective on consciousness has been supported by the teachings of science for almost one hundred years.

The quantum world — now the accepted model of reality — was opened like Pandora's box in the first half of the twentieth century by Planck, Einstein, Bohr, Heisenberg, Fermi, and Schrödinger, among others. It changed everything. No longer could the universe be understood solely in classical physics. That had done well to describe the nature of the universe and behavior of solid matter, but it could not account for the behavior of matter and energy on the subatomic scale. In 1900 Max Planck presented the idea that energy existed in individual units called "quanta," and that these units behaved in a completely new manner, which seemed to contradict the laws of physics as they had been known. Nothing is solid; everything is energy, behaving in ways that defy logic and reason. So sweeping were these discoveries that the London Times, on November 7, 1919, ran the headline: "Revolution in Science. New Theory of the Universe! Newtonian Ideas Overthrown."[83]

Planck's discovery didn't change the game as much as anticipated; here we are, nearly a century later, still acting as if the old rules of reality are the only rules. Yes, Newtonian or classical physics explains well macroscopic reality, but what and who we are as conscious beings doesn't function at that level. It is quantum theory that provides researchers with a model and language that explains the bizarre and mystical world of nonlocal mind, psychic phenomena, and life beyond death. After four hundred years of classical physics, it can be difficult to embrace the implications the quantum model makes on the very nature of what it is to be alive, let alone immortal.

Consciousness is the greatest enigma. As little as we know about our universe, we know even less about consciousness. How odd that there is nothing we experience more directly yet nothing we understand less. That's because consciousness is incredibly difficult to study! Science is objective, whereas consciousness is subjective. It does not lend itself neatly to the criteria of the scientific method: empirical, measurable effects, objective replication, results found without bias.[84] Nonetheless, an explosion in the science of consciousness has recently occurred.

While these studies examine correlations between brain function and experience, they do not study cause, what has been termed "the hard problem of consciousness." How, exactly, does experience of the self arise from matter? What makes one creature conscious and another not? Or are all conscious? Some theorize consciousness is simply an emergent quality of the brain, arising from neuronal activity. Others lean toward a non-local theory of mind, in which the brain is a mediator of or conduit for consciousness. It's worth exploring some of these theories — especially when your life is on the line — because through these explorations we're actually asking a much deeper question: do I have a soul?[85]

In 1644 one man was determined to provide an emphatic yes to that question of non-material consciousness, but he could do so only through deductive reasoning. It was a period when the scientific method was transforming society, and as the genius behind analytical geometry, René Descartes was a leader in this rational revolution. He even had the foresight to see how it would lead to the dismissal of God and the rise of material reductionism, but the measures he took to prevent this unwanted effect only contributed to it. Here was a man of deep faith and brilliant science building his philosophy of mind distinct from the brain. Materialism was growing in popularity; it sought to reduce the universe to measurable components. Descartes asserted the contrary: mind was completely different from matter. While all other aspects of reality and experience could be questioned, the existence of one's thinking self could not. Consciousness, Descartes asserted, was irrefutable, and he sought to prove it through logic. His treatise on the existence of God and the journey of our souls when they are separate from our bodies suggest he was also familiar with NDEs.[86]

Among his most famous conclusions was *Cogito, ergo sum*: I think, therefore I am. In an age when all things were called into question, the universal human experience of self-awareness, the fact that you know you exist at all, was for Descartes the undeniable premise from which to begin all inquiry on the nature of reality. But his perspective was analytical and reductionist. By transforming mathematics into metaphysics, he felt he was looking into the mind of God, "the very first and highest basic principle for the Being of beings in general," but in doing so he missed including the love of God in his calculations.

And, his critics pointed out, Descartes had a problem. Philosophers would call it substance dualism. How can mind communicate with matter if the two are of completely different natures? What is the mechanism that makes this possible? It was a good point and became the blade on which Descartes's argument fell into disrepute. Material reductionism swept into favor as the core of the scientific method. Ironically, that method would lead to the very link Descartes could not provide, but it would take another three hundred years to emerge.[87]

Descartes had another problem, and as with most eccentric geniuses, it had to do with relationships. Because he aimed his theory of knowledge to be the foundation for man's conquest of nature, Descartes separated humans from their world in order to objectify it, to master it. His theology contained no compassion or deep personal connection, just as with his life. (On that note, he never did marry and was described as a cold and selfish man who enjoyed privileged years. He did have a daughter, Francine, by a servant woman, but she died at the age of six from scarlet fever.[88]) Unwittingly, this objective stance made Descartes a symbol for all that is wrong with civilization.

His fears came true. Material reductionism is now the dominant theory of the scientific worldview. And while it seals us in the coffin of mortality, it is not without its sense of meaning and wonder, or profound stewardship for the earth. Though it dismisses any notion of God, there is still room for what feels quite mystical.[89]

And yet there remains an irony, for meaning, wonder, and feelings flow from the very thing material reductionism refutes: consciousness. Even more ironic, while the physical world is experienced second-hand, via our senses, consciousness is experienced directly. Do we not, then, have more proof for the spiritual (non-material) world than the physical? Descartes was trying to drive this home by saying the only thing you know absolutely is that your consciousness exists. Doubt the opinion of others, doubt even your senses, but you cannot doubt that. And yet many do. I choose to see this doubt as a gift, for it invigorates the dispute and calls us to wrestle authentically with the ultimate questions. But while doubt is the life-breath of the scientific method, there are limits as to how far it can follow us when we lose our breath. From that point on is something you can only know first-hand.

Must one choose between spirituality and material reductionism? Is there no middle ground? Turns out there is, and it's a new spin on one of the oldest theories out there. *Panpsychism*, a philosophy which predates Plato and proposes that all matter contains some form of consciousness, has found a new name. Integrated Information Theory (IIT) explores how consciousness may be a fundamental property of the universe. Just as an electric charge is an essential aspect of atoms, consciousness could be an essential building block of nature. If so, every system is conscious, from a photon to a rock to a human to the planet itself. This doesn't imply that a photon is aware or intelligent, but that it has some element or precursor of consciousness; limited information processes equals limited consciousness.[90] While Descartes saw the spiritual and physical as qualitatively different, panpsychics see them as quantitatively different.

Fascinating implications arise from IIT, which are profoundly spiritual. Among them is the most staggering of all: God becomes an emergent property of the universe, just as consciousness becomes an emergent property of the brain. So while God may be out there, when the universe ends, God ends.

CHAPTER 14

BELIEF

You never know how much you really believe anything until its
truth or falsehood becomes a matter of life and death to you.

— C. S. LEWIS

THE BIGGEST QUESTION TO ASK IS NOT IF GOD EXISTS, BUT WHAT IS consciousness. If it is not an emergent property of the brain, then consciousness exists independent of three pounds of gray matter between our ears. It's a small step from there to conclude (or at least seriously consider) that God exists — the primal and ultimate consciousness. If so, then consciousness is the only real estate we share with God. Invest wisely!

All healthy spiritual traditions propose, in one form or another, that God not only exists, but that God is love. So, the next question becomes personal: not Do you believe, but, How do you love. Even more, are you so audacious as to identify yourself as a manifestation of Divine Love? Are you immortal? That's the scandal of faith, not in the humility that causes one to kneel before ultimate holiness but in the boldness to stand before it, confident that you are a sacred manifestation of it.

Many of my patients would like to think they are immortal, that they will continue. They just don't want to die in order to realize it. They are filled with an understandable hope that feels frail and desperate. This hope is not grounded in identification with Divine Love, but in the deep longing to simply feel safe. And no wonder; the distress of cancer can derail efforts to form a new, coherent concept of God beyond a Sunday school faith. Even more frustrating, the hard truth is that such efforts are futile. We cannot come to know God through rational, intellectual ascent. We cannot even encounter the Divine through an emotional, heartfelt decision. Any such shift in our soul can only be in response to God already making the first move.

Edwin Abbott illustrated this nicely in a story called *Flatland*. Written in 1884, it explores what would happen if a character (a square), living in a two-dimensional reality, was visited by a sphere from a three-dimensional reality, which he cannot comprehend even as it reveals itself to him. All he sees is a circle gradually increasing, and then decreasing in size as it passes through the two dimensions. Understanding is acquired only when the square visits the three-dimensional realm.[91] Entities existing in a universe that is a subset of another cannot conceive of the nature of that higher realm by the same rules which govern the lower. So, too, we mortals can only comprehend the immortal if the immortal first reveals itself to us, and this happens through the most fundamental connection we share: love itself. Which means faith is not something we are able to come to ourselves, it is given to us. Faith is a gift. Any action on our part is a response.

Sure doesn't feel like that. Feels instead like something we need to work at (which we can), something we need to perfect (never happens), something that needs to be so strong that cancer cannot shake it. "If only I have enough faith!" (As if there was a dosage!) That statement is really a longing to feel safe in the care of a loving presence more powerful than the cancer. And in that longing is the key: only love can make us feel truly safe, for in it we are truly home.

While we cannot initiate contact with God, we certainly can tune into the distinctly spiritual abilities of consciousness, such as psychic phenomena. Unlike the small studies on Therapeutic Touch, thousands of excellent studies have been published in scientific journals, conclusively demonstrating the reality of psychic ability,[92] to the point that Jessica Utts of the

University of California, a panel member with the American Institute of Research, stated in an address to the United States Congress that it has been overwhelmingly proved to exist, and any further research should go into how it can be useful.[93]

One study has been ongoing since 1998, exploring how our interconnectivity appears to be part of the fabric of reality and is amped up considerably by strong emotion. The research was hosted by Princeton University and was running smoothly when the unthinkable happened.

It's called the Global Consciousness Project.[94] Sixty-six random number generators were placed around the globe, each one a tiny computer flipping arbitrarily between one and zero. As the data flowed to the university, researchers watched for the effect of a wonderful event that happens every year. The World Day of Prayer is held on the first Friday in March, and brings hundreds of thousands of hearts together, focused through compassion on peace. Could the energy of this intention affect the field of chaos and result in synchronizing the number generators? Sure enough, it did: minor, just a blip, but significant enough to warrant further investigation.

So the experiment continued as world events unfolded. When there was an event that caused a global emotional ripple, there, again, would be a small blip of coherence. And then, two things happened. Diana, Princess of Wales, was killed in a car accident. The ripple of grief resulted in a spike of random numbers suddenly aligning. An even greater spike occurred on 9/11. The generators began to synchronize a few minutes before the planes hit the towers. Was this the passengers realizing their fate? So powerful was the impact on people's hearts around the globe that the devices continued to synchronize for two days afterwards.[95] For over fifteen years now, data has been streaming in every second, monitoring the heartbeat of global consciousness. The odds against chance explaining the results are more than a trillion to one.

Spiritual versus material … if belief really is about a relationship, a connection, then all the intellectual tussling in the world will be fruitless. The conclusion to this argument must do more than bring peace of mind. It must bring peace to the heart, if it is to mean anything at all. For when we stand at the edge of life, dying from cancer or losing a loved one to it, the hope that we continue not only opens us to the meaning we have yet to discover on the other side, it also gives this life meaning far beyond the good we have brought to the world. All the same, the eternal significance we have in this universe starts with the temporal significance we have on this Earth. That is as noble a place to start and end a life as any. I encourage you not to settle for believing in God. I encourage you to believe *into* God, and do that through your love, even if you are dying ... especially if you are dying, for this has the power to transform you in a way that is nothing short of miraculous.

On the Edge of Immortality

THE HAIL MARY PASS. THAT'S WHAT A POORLY MATCHED UNRELATED BONE marrow transplant is — a long shot. And Brenda was going for the longest Hail Mary we'd ever seen.

Her leukemia had been very aggressive, resistant to chemo, and spreading quickly. She had no time to harvest healthy stem cells and no siblings from whom to draw that biological miracle. The only option was a MUD, but there was no time to find a match that met all ten of the HLA protein markers. The closest we could find was far below optimal, but when a 6/10 on a MUD is all you have, you really begin to consider the Hail Mary pass. It looks better than certain death; at least, it does at the beginning, especially when you're Brenda, a mom in her thirties with two young children and all of life ahead.

My first visit with her was remarkable. Enabled by the grace of the encounter and the gift of her amazing spirit, our conversation went quickly to the worst-case scenario.

"I don't think I'm going to die, even though the odds are against me." Something in the tone of her voice, the quality of her presence, made that statement resonate with conviction from a deep knowing.

"You say that with such clarity. Why is that?"

"Well, I'll tell you, and I haven't mentioned this to anyone else, not even my husband. But I had an experience. It was just the other night. I've been thinking about it ever since." My ears began to tingle.

"I was lying here, and the room was suddenly filled with this presence. Amazing peace, amazingly deep and knowing. And there was this light … the air in here changed with it. I don't know how to explain it, other than the presence of God. It was beautiful. I felt so clear about what lies ahead."

I paused. "What lies ahead …"

"Yes, how this is going to work out just fine. I don't need to be afraid. I'm not alone, and even if my body suffers, I'm going to come through this. Even …" She hesitated, as if giving herself permission to say the words. "Even if I die."

"Have you ever felt this before?"

Now she paused. Slowly, a look of recognition came upon her face. Her eyes welled up. "Yes. Yes! When my first daughter was born. It was a difficult delivery, touch-and-go for a while … I felt that same peace come over me, and I knew I would survive. It was the same presence!"

"So, it was for love that you were to remain, for the love of your child, and the one to come after. Your growth here in love was not complete."

She was weeping with awareness. "But does that mean if I die, then it's because my growth in love is complete?"

Now my turn to pause. "I wonder if it's ever complete. I wonder if it continues after. I hope so."

"Me, too."

My last visit with Brenda was equally humbling, equally inspiring. Her skin was now amber, indicating her kidneys and liver were on the verge of collapse. Jaundice first appears in the eyes, the whites turning yellow. Then the skin follows along with lethargy and confusion as carbon dioxide builds in the blood. It was to the point now that even her tears were yellow, streaking from eyes that had clouded over as her corneas disintegrated. Her skin was peeling and weeping from her body, large sections wrapped in gauze to absorb the fluid from burst capillaries. Sores filled her mouth and extended down her throat, through her entire digestive tract. Her bowels were constantly flowing.

The sight of this for nurses is very difficult. It can leave one feeling help-less. Excellent care and compassion are not enough to assuage the heart, which must break. It is all the worse for loved ones. Yet through them we have witnessed such presence, such beauty as they remain with the suf-fering. Their love becomes stronger than their fear or their helplessness.

I called upon that strength from God as I sat at her side and paused once again. What can one say? The truth. "And so it's happening."

"Yes," she whispered.

It's critical to assess physical distress first — one cannot care for the soul unless first addressing the body. "How is your pain, out of ten?"

"Fifteen." I glanced at the bags hanging from the IV pole. Dilaudid, a strong narcotic, but at what dosage?

"And, is it everywhere?"

She nodded.

"Are you afraid?"

"No, not of dying. I'm looking forward to that. It will be a release. I know where I'm going."

"And who would you like to be here when you die?" The questions are blunt because she doesn't have much time, and if the meds need to be increased to alleviate her suffering, this may be the last chance to talk and record her wishes for end-of-life care.

"My husband ..."

"How about your kids? Have you talked with them?"

"Yes, I've said all I need to say. I don't want them here. It's done." Tears quietly flowed, amber trails staining the pillow.

"Do you want to be awake or asleep when it happens?"

"Asleep."

"That will likely be the case, because there's no need for you to be suf-fering pain like this. I'd like to check with the nurse and see what can be done. It would mean increasing your Dilaudid; you'd fall asleep here and wake up there. Would that be all right?"

"Yes." It was her first smile in a long time.

"Are you afraid to fall asleep, knowing you will die?"

"No. It's OK."

Silence. Hold this reality. Hold the space. Never speak unless you can improve upon silence.

"Do you remember the feeling that you spoke of when we first met, the presence of God?"

She smiled a second time. "God seems far away, but not for long now."

I thought to myself, This would be an appropriate time to take off my shoes. Holy ground. "No, not for long. A few hours, perhaps. I think you'll see Him soon, and you will dance. You will be free. And, you'll watch over your daughters. Try not to interfere too much."

We both laughed. It is a beautiful, amazing thing to hear a dying person laugh. But she also winced. Laughter exercises your insides, and hers were in no state for a workout.

"I'm going to go check with your nurse. Let's get you comfortable."

"Thank you so much, Dave. Thank you for talking about it. It really helps."

"Thank you."

Normally I would pray, but it didn't seem as important as alleviating her pain. Her soul was at peace. God needed no request from us for that. The rest was in our hands.

Some days really fall together — the right people at the right place for the conversation. At the nursing station were the pharmacist and her nurse. We discussed pain control, called the doctor who arrived within a minute, and revised Brenda's care. She had made it clear not to have any heroic medical intervention, but to let death come naturally. Her husband was relieved with the decisions, and the meds were increased.

There's a strong desire at this point to remain. A person is about to die; it's the most critical and significant point in life. In a few hours, Brenda would undergo the transformation from this realm to the next, her consciousness shifting from the containment of the body to the limitless flight into mystery. But that would be hours away, and the reality is that there are others suffering. My care was needed elsewhere. Wrestling that desire not to miss this most important event of her life, I felt the weight of death move into me, and then the awareness that I had done all I needed to do. She was at peace. She was prepared.

But we were not. It was now the pharmacist, the doctor, the nurse, and I who quietly wept as we discussed increasing her medication, saying goodbye, and watching her slip into the dark of sleep. There is no better care than that infused with compassionate grief, the honoring of our own humanity in letting the pain flow. Grief shared is half as heavy, and we would have missed a golden opportunity if we had shrunk back from the communion before us. I sat with gratitude for our team as we drank from the cup of sorrow through being honestly and vulnerably present to each other. It was a tribute to Brenda's beautiful spirit, and to our own. In that moment we felt fully broken — and fully alive.

Brenda died that evening, comfortable and quiet in medicated sleep, her husband and the nurse at her side. Their hearts were filled with the strange harmony of gratitude and grief. I'm told the sorrow of losing his beloved, and the smile of realizing her freedom, played out upon her husband's face as he watched her breathing slow, fade, and slip away. He sat for hours afterwards, taking that rare opportunity most shy away from to contemplate life and death, the brief journey of love, and the wilderness that follows.

I TOOK A LONG WALK THAT NIGHT. I THOUGHT ABOUT HOW A SINGLE LIFE could ripple out to affect so many. I thought about how unaware Brenda was that the love she had for her husband, daughters, and others was a manifestation of something eternal, foundational, invisible. The divine consciousness that sustained her in every moment had now received her. What was it like from her side now? What was she experiencing? What wonders and perspectives was she exploring, not only about herself, but everything?

I stood under the stars once more, sending gratitude, not only for Brenda, but also for my work, and for being alive at this amazing time in human history. Here we are among the cosmos's creatures, pondering its

14 billion–year history. We are entities in a universe looking back on itself through our eyes and asking, What am I? As we gaze at those heavens, we're actually only seeing a tiny sliver of what's out there. Cosmologists tell us the physical matter that makes up "the real world" accounts for only 4 percent of the universe, and what we can see in the visible spectrum of light makes up only 0.4 percent! The rest is a mystery, which is divided into dark matter (23 percent) and dark energy (73 percent). You could think of our universe as a solitary light atop the mast of a single ship sailing upon the surface of a vast ocean: that light is the known universe, the ship is dark matter, and the ocean is dark energy. Realizing this, the hubris of the materialist scientific perspective — in thinking consciousness is an illusion of the brain — is, to me, astonishing. I could be sure it would make Brenda laugh.

The issue is really not one of science versus spirituality, but of scientism, a rigid philosophy of materialism masquerading as science. This is explored well by Professor Charles Tart, author of *The End of Materialism*.[96] He manages a website called the Archives of Scientists' Transcendent Experiences, a "safe place" for scientists to record and share their mystical experiences. Tart addresses (with considerable humor!) the cultural skepticism that refutes paranormal phenomena as a sign of a deluded mind, pointing out how a growing number of researchers are applying the scientific method and leading us to a greater understanding of the spiritual dimension of what it is to be human. To deny or suppress this is to actually inflict the greatest injury to our development as individuals, and as a species, for it seeks to undermine the very foundation and source of reality. No correlation has been found between dissociative behavior or delusional states and belief in psychic ability. In fact, there is a strong correlation between the ability to mentally focus and to experience paranormal phenomena. Rather than the result of mental deficiency, it's an aspect of mental acuity.[97] How much more important it is, then, to have an intelligible model of spirituality, one that integrates the energies of consciousness with the insights of science and the experience of humanity through all ages.

I would be remiss not to mention the insight of a friend of mine, Nina

Denham, on this subject. Nina was instrumental in refining my musings before publication. She proposed a concise corollary: At the quantum level, everything in the world is a form of energy, and all energy is information. The universe, then, is composed of just two elements: consciousness and information. Consciousness acts as a nucleus, enfolded in a field of information. What if the primary task and means of the universe's evolution is the absorption of more information by means of experience? And what if the absorption of all the information results in unity of consciousness with the Divine? Is this the grand experiment? I would propose so, and that the process and the product which result are exactly what Rene Descartes missed: love.

Fortunately, the grace of God will meet us more than halfway when we, too, struggle and stumble in love. We don't need to be perfect on this side, because we will have eternity to keep practicing on the other. I know this because I have the unique privilege of speaking with people every month who've had a look and come back to tell me about it. I know this, because their stories make me homesick for what I saw, so many years before.

PART 4

Near-Death Experiences:
The Journey Ends Well

CHAPTER 15

FOURTH TUMOR

You fainted and I caught you. It was the first time I'd supported a human. You had such heavy bones. I put myself between you and gravity. Impossible.
— ELIZABETH KNOX, *THE VINTNER'S LUCK*

THERE'S AN ANGEL STANDING ACROSS FROM ME. I CAN'T SEE IT, though I try, but the woman beside me can, and she is sobbing in wonder and awe. I had arrived at a Therapeutic Touch retreat. For two days we meditated, attended workshops, and practiced the healing art under the direction of a gifted teacher and nurse. After the second day's lecture, we divided into pairs to give and receive treatments, and I was fortunate to receive one from our teacher. Lying back on the table, I closed my eyes and prepared for what, I expected, would be the typical experience of falling into deep relaxation. What followed, though, was anything but typical.

Her hands scanned a few inches above my head, chest, and abdomen, then paused over my belly. "What's this?" she asked quietly.

"A tumor," I whispered. She stood silently over the site, focusing to detect the biofield's qualities. The treatment continued with gentle brushing gestures as she worked with my energetic anatomy. I lay still, eyes closed, feeling the weight of my body press into the table, the subtle tingle from the flow of energy moving against skin. I don't know how much time passed, but I became aware of someone quietly weeping. I opened my eyes.

The teacher stood gazing at the other side of the table. Her hands were no longer moving; she seemed paused in time as tears streamed down her face.

"What's wrong?" I asked.

She took a deep breath before reverently answering, "There's an angel of the Most High across from me. It's beautiful." I looked to the other side, excitedly anticipating an apparition of light, a vision of holiness, a glimpse of a feather, anything, anything at all. What I saw was the wall. Nothing there. I looked back to her.

She stood silent for some time, and then said, "It's gone."

Gone! Did I miss it? Was I ever meant to see it? "Well, they don't show up without a reason," I said. What little I knew of angelic appearance from my biblical studies told me they were beings of a different level of consciousness than ours, and they were messengers. To an elderly Abraham one announced he would be blessed with a child; to Elijah one gave nourishment; to the shepherds a chorus announced the birth of Christ; to Jesus they gave comfort. There are over 270 references to angels in the scriptures, and I was quite aware of the audacity of thinking I could be added as the recipient of such care. Still, I had to ask.

"What's the message?"

"He said, 'It's going to be very difficult this time, but we'll give you strength.'"

Not the most comforting announcement. Yet, I neither recoiled at what catastrophe might befall me, nor responded in praise at the promise of such care. Instead, I burst into laughter. Giggles bubbled up from my belly and curled me into a fetal position, leaving me weeping with abandon until I fell asleep. Though an odd response, it was as if I were being tickled, as if playful love had enveloped me, saying "Cheer up! It's all going to be OK."

I awoke hours later, rose from the table, stretched, and explored. The building was quiet. The encounter seemed a dream, so I grabbed my coat and walked in the late-November light along a path — a Via Dolorosa winding from the garden into the woods. This is a powerful tool for meditating upon the suffering of Christ, marked by images depicting the path Jesus walked on the way to the cross. I paused in front of each one, gazed at the reliefs, and breathed in the cold air.

At the fifth station, I paused. The image depicted Simon of Cyrene, a man who observed Jesus stumble as he carried his cross. Simon was enlisted by the soldiers to carry it for him. As I thought of the imagery — assistance coming as Jesus struggled — a large, green unopened pine cone dropped at my feet. This is me, I thought. This message said I was not finished. Like this pine cone, I was yet to open. There was still work to be done, a plan to be fulfilled. And I would receive assistance to carry my cross. Placing the pine cone in my pocket, I returned to the retreat center to thank our teacher and to ask her to describe the angel in more detail. She simply said it was a profoundly beautiful presence, astonishingly tall, and that she felt so privileged to be a part of an amazing moment. I promised to keep in touch, to let her know how I received angelic strength, then left feeling calm and excited. I pondered the experience for weeks afterwards, but told no one.

CODE BLUE

THROUGHOUT THAT YEAR I COLLAPSED ONLY A FEW TIMES. MY ABILITY to regulate my autonomic nervous system had improved, and I was no longer hesitant to step back from parish responsibilities when the tumor awoke from its slumber. Catecholamine levels had reached their highest yet, 2,500, which is five times the normal limit.

Preparing for surgery was, by now, a familiar protocol. The week to lower my blood pressure was spent chatting with other patients, watching movies, moving carefully about the unit until I could move no more. Then, we were ready. It's not uncommon to give patients something to relax before going to the operating room. I was given Valium and recall the power of this drug to turn me into the best comedian on the planet.

At least I thought so, laughing hysterically at my own puns while being wheeled on the stretcher to the OR. I regained enough composure to say another silent prayer before going to sleep.

Hours later, I awoke in intensive care for the week of observation and recovery. It was here that my assistance would come, though from my perspective, it was the medical team that needed help, not me. So I decided to give it to them.

The alarms went off at 4:00 a.m. Code blue — someone was in cardiac arrest. Poor chap, I thought, I hope they get the crash cart to him in time. And then it came crashing through my door! The medical team swarmed in with it, quickly checking monitors, blood pressure, shining lights in my eyes.

"David! David! How are you feeling?"

"Just fine. How are you?"

The nurse paused, looked at me. Clearly she was expecting a different response.

"What's going on?" I asked.

"Your blood pressure's gone down; we're just going to stabilize it."

"Mm-hmm," I responded while watching tubes, lines, and machines appear around me. I looked up at the young doctor. "Hello."

His glare told me he had no time for such pleasantries. "Stats!" he barked.

"BP ... Systolic 80, temp 37.7, pulse 130, 140." The numbers, I would later learn, indicated a lack of arterial pressure. Despite my heart furiously pounding away as it tried to force blood through my body, the veins and arteries had lost their ability to constrict, leaving my blood to settle and pool.

A nurse continued to read off numbers, "CVP 10, systolic now 70." My central pressures were not improving. Cardizem and metoprolol, drugs to prevent heart attack, were injected. No change.

"Dopamine 10mcg."

"BP now 100 systolic." Not much of a change. Saline and Pentaspan were pushed to increase blood volume, but it was the dopamine that should have boosted my pressure by causing the blood vessels to constrict, forc-ing the pressure back up. It did nothing.

"Damn. It's not working," the doctor said, his mind clearly racing to the next step. "Somebody call his wife."

That was not comforting.

"We have to check his heart. I'm going to use a Swan-Ganz."

I smiled as the nurse swabbed my neck. Her eyes darted to her col-leagues, back to me, tension written all over her face.

"David, I have to put a line into your heart," the doctor said. "There's going to be a pinch at your neck." The Swan-Ganz is a catheter threaded through a vein into the upper chamber of the heart, which allows the doc-tor to monitor the heart's function, pressure, and blood flow. The situation was critical. It was clear they were frantically trying to avert a catastrophe, but I seemed oblivious to the distress.

I simply said, "OK." Didn't feel the scalpel slice open the vein, didn't feel the thick line snaking through my neck and chest as the doctor tried to feed it to the correct section of the heart, his eyes fixed on the monitor.

"Damn! Damn! It's gone in wrong. I have to do it again."

I gazed reassuringly at the doctor. Clearly he was frazzled. It would be a shame for him to get even more worked up.

"You look stressed," I said. "I'll sing you a song." And then one of my favorite hymns came to mind, "Spirit of Gentleness." I happily hummed away while the medical team stared in disbelief. Here I was going through cardiac crisis but acting like I was getting a manicure. I honestly did not know what came over me (well, I did later).

Fortunately, the doctor was successful in placing the second line. It didn't take long for the readings to confirm their suspicions. The heart's SVR, or systemic vascular resistance, should have been 800-1200, mine was 322. My heart rate was also going up to compensate, trying to push more fluid to the organs, but my blood was barely flowing. Cardiac out-put should have been 12, but it dropped to 2.

The issue was a drug given during surgery to lower my blood pressure enough to give plenty of headroom when the tumor blew during removal.

Phenoxybenzamine is an alpha-adrenergic blocker used for hypertension. It had been very effective, helping me avert death at the most critical time in the surgery. Ironically, residual elements of it were now threatening me, and what I needed at this point was the very stimulant my tumor had used to put my life in danger: norepinephrine. It would constrict the blood vessels even further, pulling me out of the nosedive.

"Levophed!" This was the norepinephrine, which the nurse hung as a drip beside the saline. The team watched the monitors, and I watched the team, happily humming along. The readings began to shift, the Swan-Ganz recording an increase in arterial tension. Heart rate 85, blood pressure 115/55. Veins and arteries were tightening up. Pressure returned to normal, and a sigh of relief from the doctor told me that he would, too. The team cleared up their mess and faded back to the unit, leaving me to twiddle my toes and nap.

Early that morning, at the end of the shift, one of the nurses came and sat by my side. "All right, young man, what the hell was that?"

"What was what?"

"That singing and humming and all your niceness. You were in cardiac arrest! Numbers through the bottom! We stuck a line in your heart and pumped you up with drugs we never give to conscious patients! Most don't wake up from an episode like that!"

I shrugged, feeling a bit sheepish and responsible, as if I had caused a lot of unnecessary bother. "I just thought you all looked a bit stressed, thought I'd try to calm you down."

I had no recollection of the angelic message given weeks before, until I was well into my recovery at home. It left me feeling like the dimmest bulb in the drawer, but also deeply grateful. *It's going to be very difficult this time, but we'll give you strength.* I marveled at how gentle that strength was. The peace had quietly flowed into me, enveloping me with a light-hearted playfulness and gentle comfort. *It's going to be OK.*

CHAPTER 16

NEAR-DEATH EXPERIENCES

The phoenix must burn to emerge.

— JANET FITCH, *WHITE OLEANDER*

VISIONS OF THE UNDISCOVERED COUNTRY EXTEND BACK THOUSANDS of years. They are found in the Bible, *The Tibetan Book of the Dead*, and in Plato's *Republic*. They permeate the *Upanishads* and the sacred texts of ancient Babylon. They flow through the poetry of the *Tao Te Ching*, and are depicted in the art and stories of pre-Columbian American cultures. Every period has its version of the mystic realm. No religion or people are alone in attempting to portray that wonder.

The modern age is also replete with accounts of the afterlife, even more so as technology enables us to snatch the soul back from the brink. While statistics as to how often this occurs hover around 10 percent for cardiac patients,[98] that can rise to 30 percent for people during other events that are not life-threatening, such as during childbirth, accidents, surgery, and illness.[99] This aligns with my own experience, for due to the nature of my job I hear of accounts every month. Some are current, some are retrospective from years before, even from childhood. All are marked with a strange mixture of conviction and bewilderment.

Lisa's story is typical, if such a word can be used to describe the phenomenon! "I had been struggling with an infection," she related. "They said that was common with chemo, but I never expected it to be so bad, fever of 104, shaking all over. I was delirious, with weird dreams. Then, one night it got really rough. I was looking at the nurse, when the room seemed to close in around me and I passed out. Suddenly I'm looking at myself from above, yet I felt really calm. They were working on my body. I wasn't afraid. It was like I didn't care. Then this light drew me in and it was … it was …" Lisa paused, staring at the blanket as the memory filled her. Her eyes brimmed with tears, then turned to me as she sobbed the words. "It was beautiful!"

I deliberately held the space so the experience could surface like a sunken treasure emerging from the depths. She began to smile. "I've never felt so happy. This light was all around me, this love beyond anything I've known." She shook her head. "I completely forgot about the cancer, the hospital, my life here. There was only the light and me." She paused, smile fading. "Then I was back. It seems so far away now." Her tears fell softly, the room imbued with sadness and wonder.

"I woke in the ICU with all these machines around me. I felt so small."

"Did you tell the nurse?" I asked.

"No, no. I haven't told anyone but my husband. It seems strange, but I'm not afraid anymore. What was it? A hallucination?"

"Well, how does it compare with any hallucinations or dreams you've had before?"

"Oh, not the same," she said. "No, this was … this was more real. This was so good. I feel this. I know this."

Lisa did well through the rest of her treatment, and left with a secret smile upon her soul, now one among millions who've been temporarily transformed. But she also left troubled, out of sorts. While elated that she'd walked heaven's shore, in a way she felt more lost than ever.

How could this be? It sounds like such a desirable experience. You'd think anyone would be overjoyed to have humanity's hope directly confirmed. But it leaves you homesick and confused. It leaves you secretly aching to be seized again by such love and made whole, to be one with the song of life. That realm interrupts your comfortable distraction, your half-hearted awareness. It can introduce profound existential tension. Realizing how impoverished your state, you are hungry for heaven, and nothing on earth satisfies. The poets express this best. Thoreau wrote of it in "Inspiration" while in seclusion at Walden Pond:

> I hear beyond the range of sound,
> I see beyond the range of sight,
> New earths, and skies and seas around,
> And in my day the sun doth pale his light.

No wonder we question its veracity. So utopian is the vision that many see it only as wish fulfillment to compensate for what has been, throughout the span of time, an astonishing struggle: humanity's climb toward the thin veneer of civilization that lies upon a deep history of violence, brutality, and survival of the fittest. Surely, heaven must be evolution's Prozac, a development of the brain to compensate for our unique ability to realize our mortality. Such is the conclusion of material reductionism as it seeks to refute the growing evidence that points to a land beyond this corporeal realm. The resistance is understandable. After all, the phenomena of NDEs change the whole game of who and what we are, and do not lend themselves to the scientific method. Can it ever affirm what has been held throughout the course of time: that death is but a pause, a comma, not a period?

Scientific theories chalk NDEs up to end-of-life metabolic processes, such as cerebral hypoxia (loss of oxygen to the brain), hypercarbia (increased carbon dioxide in the brain), endorphins, or a final burst of electrical activity in the brain. Or are NDEs merely a psychological phenomenon, a dissociative defense mechanism to cushion the final blow? Let's look at the arguments, present some possibilities, and, hopefully, add some original insights to the wise and experienced authors who have written volumes on the ultimate mystery of life: whether it continues.

Going down this road does not mean you're giving up! But we have to explore this if we are to truly engage with the spiritual journey of cancer. Most people do this privately, anxiously and sporadically, wary of "feeding" cancer with negative energy. How much better to contemplate death with curiosity, wisdom, and acceptance. After all, your eventual passing is inevitable, and you are complex enough to hold life and death in your heart at the same time. In fact, doing so has the surprising effect of making life even better, since you're no longer straining against this fundamental aspect of your humanity. So, first step is some basic orientation.

NDEs were brought into popular culture in 1975, with Raymond Moody's *Life After Life*. While his definition and identifying markers held true for years, subsequent research reveals considerable variety in NDEs.[100] They are as unique as each individual, which should be no surprise. The mind is astonishingly complex; how much more so the soul and the web of ego-identification we build around it.

Researchers look for NDEs with specific markers. They want a verified clinical death, patients must be unconscious with fixed dilated pupils, they must have stopped breathing, and their brains must be anoxic. Cut off from oxygen for even thirty seconds, the brain begins to die. That is significant, especially as there are many cases of NDE in which the brain has been deprived of oxygen for minutes, even hours. Of course, most NDEs do not occur under such measurable conditions. Those are helpful if you're exploring the process of death, but not so much if you're interested in the experience of death itself.

One quality commonly shared is what Lisa struggled with as we explored her experience: ineffability. When you've visited a realm so different from this, words simply fail to describe what you've seen. Integrating an alternate dimension is no small feat, which is why for many, it remains buried in the subconscious, taking years to recall and a lifetime to integrate.

In many cases the experiencer knows they are dead, yet they are not disturbed by this change, as was the case with Lisa. She saw the medical team try to revive her, and the nurse later verified that her heart had stopped. This awareness is sometimes marked by disorientation, fear, and a delay in recognizing one's own body, but most feel a compassionate detachment, as Lisa did. One person, on recounting their NDE, said with a smile, "Death is the safest thing you could ever go through." That was an astonishing thing to hear, and I was glad for him, but as we will see, it may not be so safe for everyone.

Lisa also had an out-of-body experience (OBE). More commonly reported in Western cultures, these are valuable to researchers in that the individuals are sometimes able to report activity, conversations, and details in the room when they should be dead, or very close to it. Even more astonishing is when they accurately report on what loved ones are doing down the hall, or hundreds of miles away.[101]

Other beings are sometimes encountered, which only make sense if consciousness is, indeed, the foundation of reality. We call them angels, though their variety may be more diverse than imagined. These entities radiate immense power, wisdom, and compassion and are distinctly different from the spirits of loved ones. While human souls can, along with other celestial beings, appear as luminescent forms, they often are recognizable as the people you've known. And they look great, radiating vitality and joy. To be received by those who would make you feel most safe is a great comfort when you contemplate your inevitable journey to the afterlife.

A fascinating aspect in some accounts is music. This is so much more than a good tune. It is heard in the soul and is infused with what can only be described as praise. Everything, survivors report, is kept in place by this vibration from God. The sacred geometry of sound is the divine instrument of creation.[102]

Then there is that presence, an astonishingly transcendent and omnipotent Being. This Consciousness is called by many names: the Higher Self, Ultimate Awareness, the Source, and of course, God. Attempts to describe this are replete with superlatives, yet since this presence emanates such supernatural compassion, intelligence, and omnipotence, words become barren and empty. Repeatedly, experiencers are left, as Lisa was, struggling to describe the indescribable. Her tears were more accurate than any verbal depiction could be.

There are many NDEs that include a life review. You are shown how every facet of your life either contributed to love's advancement or held it back. This is presented with no judgment, only a desire that you be completely authentic and aware of how your choices affected your growth in love and that of others. Most bracing is that experiencers report feeling every moment of their life again *from the perspective of everyone they influenced* — the whole ripple effect. Here one judges oneself. I can think of no greater evaluation than to stand naked before the great cosmic mirror, and hope I can be half as compassionate with my flaws as the heavenly hosts around me.

If it feels the weight of your sins tips the scales as you imagine this, the best response is the honest remorse so many feel during the life review — but don't stay there, beating yourself up! This is an opportunity to grow, not to recycle the pain for eternity. Lord knows, we do enough of that here! Brené Brown speaks to this in her wonderful TED Talk, Listening to Shame:

> Guilt is saying, I did something bad. Shame says, I am something bad.... Guilt: I'm sorry. I made a mistake. Shame: I'm sorry. I am a mistake.[103]

It's nothing new: contrition, remorse, confession, apology, restoration, healing. We're called to get real and grow. In this way we use our failings as fuel to fly higher.

Which brings us to advanced experiences. These become even more transcendent, with visions of communities in which beings live, creating and contributing to a culture of continued experience, a place where no one sits idle with a harp on a cloud. All seem involved in the continued evolution of their souls, learning, growing, practicing new skills, and expressing that through art, music, study, cooperative projects, and play. We may have a busy life waiting, one connected fully with our ability to contribute as unique expressions of God's love. I wonder if this will even include playing a part in the administration and care of the universe. Are these images real or projections of consciousness tailored to the individual's ability to understand? That remains to be seen, but what is clear is that wonders await us.[104]

Many experiencers come to a barrier of some kind. This may be a visible structure such as a fence or door, a natural formation like a river, or it may simply be a point at which one cannot continue. While some are given a choice, others are told they must return to continue their growth in love. That return to the body is a difficult and disheartening experience, so limiting and sluggish compared to the expansive state of consciousness they had on the other side.

Remarkably, NDEs can also be shared. Those in the presence of the dying can experience the initial stages of the transformation. They, too, describe rising out of their bodies, seeing the spirit of their loved one, hearing heavenly music, observing their loved one's life review, seeing deceased relatives and transcendent beings.[105] I have spoken with several nurses over the years who recall a shift in the light and energy in the room when a patient dies, and I've been privileged to support family members in debriefing the experience months or even years after. While this is often very comforting, sometimes it's frightening.

One such case involved removal of life support in the intensive care unit. The patient had struggled with cancer and gone to extraordinary lengths to fight for the sake of her daughters. Now they surrounded her unconscious body in sadness, telling her it was okay to go, that they could continue without her here on earth. However, the youngest daughter, Angela, was most distressed. She had a phobia of hospitals and death ever since her own NDE during an illness years earlier. Angela remembered the fear as she separated from her body and moved toward the light. Worse was the discovery that she maintained a link to the other side: unusual psychic abilities were driving her crazy. It's not uncommon for these to increase as we approach death, but they can be among several unexpected side effects of returning from it.[106]

As she shared her story with me, I was able to explain how common this was, that heightened psychic ability was part of the development of her consciousness, and that her OBE was the initial stage of what, eventually, will be a grand adventure. Normalizing this empowered Angela to stay at the bedside as her mother's breath faded. Then Angela turned pale and gripped my hand. "I can see her spirit rising from her body," she whispered.

I calmly guided her ability. "Send her love. Send her a thank you for being your mom. Send your blessing as she goes."

The energy in the room seems to shift, then return to normal, as did Angela. She felt oddly peaceful, instead of simply odd. Talking her through this as it occurred, with her sisters listening, was critical in repairing her frightening OBE experience, and in helping her manage her increased psychic awareness. I also gave her resources to help process what had happened years earlier — positive first steps in living with a heightened state of consciousness.

Group experiences occur when two or more people die and participate together in the phenomena. While rare, group NDEs contain spectacular details, as the experiencers see each other leave their bodies, then share messages and observations while still experiencing the near-death state. Upon revival, they are shocked and comforted to find their experiences align.

An excellent example of this was told by May Eulitt to her physician, Dr. Stephen Hoyer.[107] She and her cousin James and his friend Rashad were electrocuted by a lightning bolt, which struck a metal gate they were all touching. Suddenly, they found themselves in a large stone hall. At the end was a lighted archway, through which they entered a breathtaking vista of meadows, hills, and mountains. Each of them saw this according to their own cultural filters: to May it was heaven, to James, the Gulf of Souls, and to Rashad, Nirvana.

An angelic being appeared, again interpreted uniquely: for May she was a guardian name Helena, for James it was his deceased father, and for Rashad, the Buddha. They were shown how their friendship helped shape Rashad's soul, and that he would soon experience death's final transformation and enter Nirvana. The three returned with new awareness of humanity's one purpose — to love God and each other, for all living things in the universe were expressions of the One Consciousness. Details of their future were also revealed, and indeed came to pass. Rashad would die a year after his return. James would die three years later of a brain tumor, donating a considerable inheritance to a charity that educated young people in India. May would live another thirty years with this experience a guiding force in her life.

It's fascinating to see how the overall structure of an NDE remains the same throughout time and civilizations. However, as one drills down to the details of the experience, it becomes more specific according to historic period, culture, traditions, language, and finally to the personality and life story of the individual.[108] The case above is an excellent example of this. How could it be otherwise? If Yama, god of the dead from the Hindu faith, greeted me, I would not understand the meaning or significance of that being. Just as we are greeted by the souls of those we have known, so too are spiritual figures going to be the ones comprehensible to us. Author Nancy Evans Bush explains this nicely:

> The description of any NDE is dependent upon the pre-existing mental categories and vocabulary of the person doing the describing. For instance, encountered entities are not reported as introducing themselves or wearing name tags, but are identified by the experiencer according to whatever labels are present in the person's cognitive storehouse; people do not describe presences or other elements in terms that are unfamiliar to them. It may be that, especially with religious figures, identification is bound up with the content and ascribed meaning of the experience, though it cannot be confirmed as literal fact.[109]

For some Christians, this may be doctrinally very threatening as they recall the words of Jesus in John 14:6: "I am the way, the truth and the life. No one comes to the Father except through me." However, NDEs that do not include Jesus only demonstrate that experience and interpretation are specific to an individual's ability to comprehend and express them in familiar terms. It does not undermine the identity of Jesus as the way, the truth and the life. The primary message of NDEs is consistent with His teachings: we are children of God, and we are to evolve in love.[110] By tuning our consciousness to the frequency of heaven, we become instruments through which others not only hear the song, but also join that symphony. Engaging this must be specific to each individual, so it makes sense that celestial greeters are so personalized. While Jesus does show up frequently in Western NDE accounts, the other emissaries are no less endowed with His love and compassion.

We'd like to think those who have led a good life, believe in God, or have accepted Christ through a personal prayer would have only positive NDEs, while the depraved, the selfish, and the unbelieving would have negative ones. It would be comforting to have your heavenly membership so stamped and approved. However, no connection has been found between character, religious belief, age, race, sexual orientation, the means of coming close to death (including suicide)[111] and the likelihood of having a positive or distressing NDE.[112] "Good" people have had distressing ones, and "bad" people have had pleasant ones.

Distressing experiences seem to fall into three categories: Inverse ones have features usually reported as pleasurable or interesting, but are perceived as threatening. Void experiences are marked by a vast dark emptiness, which can be a positive experience for some, terrifying for others. The third type is just what you'd expect.[113]

Yes, visions of hell do occur, though they are the least common form of distressing NDEs. These complex events are marked not so much by physical torture as a range of distress, from painful emotion to outright spiritual agony. While there are some accounts with evil creatures and forsaken souls, the main quality of these experiences, from the few distressing NDEs known to researchers, is a sense of forsakenness rather than evil.[114] This makes sense, as the theological definition of hell is a condition of separation, not a specific place. Just as absolute zero (0˚K or -273.15˚C) is not a measurement of the intensity of cold but of the absence of heat, so hell is not a place of burning fire or unending torment, but a condition of the utter absence of the sacred.

While this may not sound as bad as eternal torture, consider that we exist in a reality that arises from the spiritual realm. St. Paul describes this sacred soup in Acts 17:28 as that through which we live and move and have our being. So immersed, we take it for granted as we do the air we breathe. Remove that air, though, and you're in trouble. Remove your being from God, and the desolation is unimaginable.

Most hellish experiences find the experiencer observing, rather than being immersed in that alternate realm. Torment may be witnessed or interpreted but is not actually felt.[115,116]

While there are a few modern cases of those who've traveled to the underworld, most accounts of a fiery realm come not from the average Joe who went south, but from those you'd imagine least likely to do so: saints, mystics, and holy people. Their tales are found in all manner of faiths throughout time, and are the most extreme example of what Joseph Campbell called the monomyth — the universal archetype of the Hero's Journey.[117] This is the process by which a person is thrown into a danger, fraught with challenges and possible destruction, yet through which they are transformed. Drawing on Jungian theory, these epic journeys to the underworld become the ultimate pilgrimage toward existential integration or disintegration, toward identifying with love or fear. Interestingly, they are prototypical of shamanic training, a transformation by fire, so to speak.

For the rest of us mortals, however, tales of hell's visitation feel anything but epic — more like a nightmare, and one that may be of our own creating. If we are what we repeat, as Aristotle said, do we build our home in hell brick by brick, with every unloving thought, word, and action? I wonder if, in the NDE life review, that pattern is laid bare to us. We realize what we have become and where we can exist. Hell, from this perspective, becomes our choice, not God's punishment. In the life review, the questions are put to us: Can you accept that you are an expression of God? That you are, and always have been, entwined with God's consciousness? That your name is love? [118] This is a truth affirmed in the Christian rite of baptism, as well as the rituals of other faiths. All that is not of love is forgiven, which is fundamentally an act of remembrance.

Put another way, the separation that comes from ego-identification is recognized as spiritual insanity. How could you ever be separate from God? As a conscious being, you have always been one with Divine Love. Any moment, with the Spirit's help, we can choose to realize that separation, however convincing it may be, is an illusion. Salvation becomes a present identity of wholeness instead of a future hope to be so healed. Of course, we don't need to wait until a life review to claim that inheritance. To walk with purposeful awareness that you are already a restored and glorious spiritual being here on Earth brings a bit of heaven to this life and helps restore the memory of it in others.

Our modern concept of hell, along with the idyllic heaven, was actually not part of Jewish culture in the time before Christ. The afterlife for them was more nuanced, with celestial realms reserved for royalty, while the rest of us went to ambiguous states of consciousness, still able to trouble our living relatives from the great beyond nonetheless. Hell, as most people think of it today, is a European model developed during the early days of Christianity to ensure the obedience of converts. The biblical term is actually "Gehenna of fire," and refers to the city dump outside Jerusalem, which also used to be a place of human sacrifice.

The word itself comes from Norse mythology and refers to Hel, the queen of the dead and ruler of "the other world." Most souls were understood to "go to Hel," and like the *bardos* or transitional stages of purification in *The Tibetan Book of the Dead*, this could be a temporary realm among many.[119] Divination and ancestral worship were common practices to appease those restless souls, even to gain their favor. Hell as a place of eternal punishment is, then, a fairly recent development in the timeline of history. I suspect it is also an aspect of our projected violence and desire for justice, as much as a metaphysical reality.

The reader may be asking at this point if I believe hell is real (if you haven't already thrown the book across the room!). The answer is a definitive yes — as real as the reality you are presently experiencing. Which is to say, not as real as you may think. (OK, throw the book.) To explain, we must leave religious concepts for a while and dive into the new mysticism: quantum physics.

It turns out that the universe is fuzzy, more a projection of consciousness than an "objective" reality.[120,121] At the smallest scale of the universe lies the quantum field, a realm of pure energetic potential in which a photon behaves like a wave. But an odd thing happens when you bring your consciousness to the field: the wave changes to behave like a particle. It's called the collapse of the wave function. Quantum energy shifts from the possible to the particular, it is concretized through consciousness into space and time. Every moment we participate in this paradox. When enough photons behave as particles and slow down to create interference patterns, you get matter (which is still mostly empty space — the void is vast between the electrons at the outer edge of the atom and the nucleus at its heart). All this is initiated by your being, your consciousness. Since the collapsed field manifests the reality you experience, it means there is no "objective" reality apart from the observer. It does not mean you alone create your reality, since we need to factor in the full spectrum of consciousness, from ants to archangels and beyond. The implication is no less staggering: this reality may be a projection from the spiritual level of pure consciousness — a hologram.[122,124] If that's the case, I see no reason why hell is not also a projection of consciousness. Perhaps we become psychically trapped in a construct defined and dominated by the darkness of our subconscious mind. Combine that darkness with the collective madness that saturates our species, and the result can only be described as hell.

Yet, all that is a puff of smoke compared to the reality of God.[125] I say this based, in part, on a reassuring nuance among distressing NDEs: there are cases when an individual in torment called out for help, and it came. An angelic figure, a divine rescuer, a guide through the madness, someone or something showed up and took the person from the distressing state to a heavenly realm.[126] Some then have a life review, and come to understand how they denied love and identified instead with fear. But this doesn't happen in all cases. There are some for whom no heavenly rescue comes, only an earthly revival, which leaves them haunted by the event. Perhaps their resuscitation interrupted the celestial intervention, resulting in a higher level of post-traumatic stress and increased fear of death from there on.

That the rescue happens at all is hopeful, and indicates that a distressing NDE may, in fact, be an incomplete NDE.[127] The experience could function as a purification process, the ultimate in hard love to wake a person up. All the more critical, then, for these individuals to seek out a therapist familiar with this esoteric phenomenon, one who can guide the survivor to deeper insights on their life, get to work on healing their relationships and their soul, and most of all, reaffirm God's absolute love.

I acknowledge the immense ambiguity of this frontier, but what does consistently emerge from NDEs (and other explorations) is the exciting perspective that consciousness is the web of Being: the universe emerges from life itself, not the other way around.[128] Which may explain why so many, on being "reunited" with that realm, describe it as home.

THE VISION OF HOME

IT WAS, FORTUNATELY IN A HOSPITAL CHAPEL THAT I DIED. THIS WAS DURing internship, before I discovered the second tumor growing on my femoral artery. I was there to do a church service for patients and staff. As on other Sundays, the cramps and sweat preceded the collapse. As on other Sundays, I breathed deep and kept on going into the sermon. And then I stopped breathing, and blacked out. I was gone before I hit the floor. What happened next was unlike any Sunday I've known, but it became the only Sunday — the only time I've truly worshiped. What I saw can only be summed up in one word: home.

A green field, a hill, the colors ... so intense, so beautiful! And the light ... the light was staggering, not in its brilliance but in its clarity, and its joy. It was saturated with joy. Light didn't emanate from a sun above, but from everywhere, from everything. The grass caressed my bare feet with each step that brought me closer to the crest of the hill. And on that crest was a singular tree, its branches stretched achingly wide to drink in the light. My heart burst with longing to reach it. Exaltation on the edge of release blocked my breath. I knew what lay beyond that tree, on the other side of that hill: it was wonder, it was adventure, it was the landscape I had longed for in the deepest dimensions of my heart. It was home.

There's no other word for it. It felt as if I had returned to a place hidden deep in my soul, and in doing so returned to myself, absolutely free, absolutely complete, and absolutely happy. My senses perceived the movement of every blade of grass, stirred by a breeze that also flowed through me with the light, and I was one with elation. Pure bliss. I laughed with the giddy excitement of a child at Christmas, and exclaimed, "I'm home! I'm home! I'm home!"

"It's good to see you, David. Welcome!" The Presence walked by my side, a profoundly gentle and loving entity who felt like my best friend, yet was also a powerful, wise, and tender guardian. I remember feeling so relaxed in His company, as if we had known each other all my life. His voice was deeply comforting, infused with authority and knowledge. I felt His words with my entire being. Yet, I did not gaze at Him; I never saw Him. If I had simply turned, He would have been there. Oddly, I didn't. I didn't care what He looked like, for I was apprehended by joy, seized by rapture, and gloriously more alive than I have ever known.

"It's so good to be here!" I exclaimed, practically bouncing with jubilation as we walked together.

"Yes, it's good to have you here. And you're doing fine, you're doing very well. However, there's a lot more work to do, so you can't stay. You have to go back."

Ridiculous, I thought. Go back? Silliest thing anyone could suggest! "Why would I go back?" I exclaimed. "I'm here, I'm home. I'm not going anywhere." Resolute, I willed my feet to continue, to run, yet His peace and clarity seemed to resign my mind to the inevitable outcome.

Again the assurance, "You're doing fine. Everything's going according to plan, but you can't stay." My heart sank, even as it was held by His astonishing compassion.

"I'm not going back there. This is what I've been waiting for." My voice was now a whisper, more breath than words: "I'm home. I'm finally home." How could I possibly arrive only to be sent back? We hadn't even reached the crest of the hill! Surely He didn't expect me to return without seeing what was on the other side? Please, please, I thought, let my eyes drink it in. Let me disappear in its beauty. My heart felt as though it would leap from my chest and race ahead of me. Longing filled my soul even as it ached to be filled. "I'm not going back. I can't go back." I felt Him smile, then heard Him laugh, warm and understanding, parental and patient, confident and clear. He laughed with tender endearment, and then gently placed His hand on my shoulder. "We'll see you later."

And that was it. Suddenly, the awful weight, the density of flesh, the hard floor against my face. My limbs weighed a ton, my mind groped through darkness and muck, smell and sound, everything fractured. Voices in the distance were calling. *Let me sleep. Let me go back.* Then I realized where I was, and my heart just broke. I cried like a child. *No, not here. Not this. So close. Why couldn't I stay? I don't want to be here. Let me go, let me go home.* I grieved like a lost lover, then instinctively buried it deep. It descended in a breath to the dark recesses of my soul. They rolled me on my back. A nurse was leaning over me; a doctor was checking my pulse.

"You OK? You know where you are?" The standard questions, again.

"Yes," I quietly said, "I know where I am. I'm in the hospital. It happened again. I'm sorry. I'm so sorry to scare everyone." I was thinking of the patients, but the nurse was scared, too, as was my wife.

"Your heart stopped, David. It was a lot worse this time. You were gone."

I didn't tell her. I didn't tell anyone. The experience was swallowed in the slow, plodding mire of ordinary moments — breathing, thinking, moving this gross form, and worst of all, communication; the sheer effort was astonishing and always inaccurate. So, I became silent, and contemplated what had seemed a dream. It must have been. It was a dream. I was taken to a clinic room. I drank the orange juice, smiled to acknowledge pleasant assurances, pulled the blanket close about my shoulders. We went home, where I slept and secretly mourned.

CHAPTER 17

HOPE, HYPOXIA, AND HYPOTHESES

Love never ends.

1 CORINTHIANS 13:8

I KNOW WHAT YOU'RE THINKING. I'VE THOUGHT IT TOO, AS I WRESTLED and wondered if the other world was real. It's all nonsense. Foolishness. There are plenty of reasonable explanations for these stories. Let's go through the list.

Hypoxia. Everyone's experienced this, the momentary drop in blood pressure that starves the brain of oxygen when you stand. I know hypoxia well, and not simply because it's a common effect of pheochomocytoma. As a really tall guy, I've earned the title "orthostatic man." This honor does not come with a cape and mask, but rather blurred vision and a nasty bump on the head. Given how quickly one feels nauseous and faint, it's no wonder even thirty seconds of oxygen starvation can leave the brain permanently damaged.

When our brains are hypoxic, several things happen that appear similar to NDEs. First is the neural noise in the eye, something called retino-cortical mapping. Combined with vascular constriction, it results in peripheral vision dropping off to a pinpoint of light surrounded by small, bright, flashing points of lights and motion. That explains zooming through a tunnel. Tachycardia (rapid heartbeat) and hypertension (high blood pressure) accompany this process, resulting in tingling and a high-pitch sound. Surprisingly, a feeling of peace is often reported with hypoxia, and one can have an out-of-body experience. Test pilots report this frequently as they spin in a centrifuge during training, causing the blood to drain from their heads. High-altitude mountaineers also experience this, along with euphoria.

Yet, there are significant differences between hypoxia and NDEs. If the tunnel experience is due to loss of peripheral vision, then this should be a universal aspect of the phenomenon. But the tunnel seems culturally specific; it is rarely reported in NDEs from Eastern societies. Tingling and an auditory buzzing are sometimes reported, but again, are not consistent qualities of NDEs. And, while OBEs are not uncommon with severe hypoxia, those individuals see themselves from a lateral perspective, while with an NDE it's most often a vertical one, floating above the scene. Also, the body is distorted with hypoxic perception, hands and head out of proportion due to the concentration of nerves in these areas. Similar effects are observed in sensory deprivation experiments. Not so with NDEs. Most significantly, the peace and euphoria of an NDE remain a permanent memory, along with details of a very complex experience. Hypoxia, on the other hand, results in fragmented thinking and loss of memory.

Further, with hypoxia, higher brain functions fail, preventing the ability to think or speak. Yet during NDEs, people try to communicate with medical staff and other individuals nearby, and have astonishing conversations with spiritual beings and deceased relatives who greet them. NDEs also can occur without hypoxia, such as during childbirth and in accidents. When the brain has been starved of oxygen during an NDE, the expected brain damage does not occur. The individual actually has enhanced memory, amazing perceptual orientation, experiences no convulsions, exhibits accelerated healing, and unlike any hallucination or delusion, an NDE results in permanent life changes. Hypoxia also cannot account for shared or group death experiences, nor explain the ability of the deceased to report what is going on in the room or details of conversations — perceptions that simply should not be possible.

Dr. Sam Parnia, assistant professor of medicine at the State University of New York and a leading researcher of NDEs among cardiac patients, comments:

> The data suggests that in [the] cardiac arrest model, the NDE arises during unconsciousness. This is a surprising conclusion, because when the brain is so dysfunctional that the patient is deeply comatose, the cerebral structures that underpin subjective experience and memory must be severely impaired. Complex experiences such as are reported in the NDE should not arise or be retained in memory. Such patients would be expected to have no subjective experience (as was the case in 88.8% of patients in this study) or at best a confusional state if some brain function is retained.[129]

One famous case illustrating the limitations of the hypoxia hypothesis involves singer-songwriter Pam Reynolds, a woman who underwent a radical, innovative procedure for a brain stem aneurysm in 1991. It remains one of the most reliable cases for scientific scrutiny, as she was rendered clinically dead under full instrumentation. Her NDE is "the single best instance we now have in the literature on near-death experiences to confound the skeptics,"[130] according to Kenneth Ring, professor emeritus of psychology at the University of Connecticut.

A mother of three small children, Reynolds was betting on the slim chance the operation offered. To prevent the blood vessel from rupturing, her body temperature was lowered to 60°F. Once cooled, the surgical table was angled so blood could be drained from her brain. There was no heartbeat, no brain activity, no sign of life. All the monitors confirmed she was dead. Yet, Pam later reported hearing the sound of the drill, then a popping sensation, and suddenly observing her operation from above the table. She noticed the surgical instrument used on her head resembled her father's Dremel tool. She saw the bits and attachments for the device. She noticed that her head had not been shaved as she expected. All the while Pam's eyes were covered and taped shut, her ears plugged with headphones that emitted a loud clicking sound to aid in registering any brain activity.

Pam found herself drawn to a light, encountered deceased relatives as well as a friend she did not know was dead. These are very complex perceptions for someone with no brain function! At one point she asked about the light, if it was God. The response: "No. The light is what happens when God breathes." I'm standing in the breath of God, she thought.[131] Despite her love for her family, she didn't want to return. It was her uncle who led her back to her body and told her to jump in. Pam resisted. She argued and negotiated and pleaded with her uncle. So astounding was this plane of consciousness, she had no hesitation in reasoning that her kids would be just fine without her. And then her uncle gave Pam a shove. She recalled the sensation was like falling into ice water and jokes that she never quite forgave him for that. The experience of such astonishing light and love left Pam forever changed.

A critical component of Pam's NDE is veridical information (information that coincides with physical reality). She reported details in her surroundings and events that occurred while she had no heartbeat or brain activity, and she reported meeting the spirit of someone she did not know was dead. These details were later verified as true.

In a 2009 review, Dr. Janice Holden, department chair of counseling at the University of North Texas and editor of the *Journal of Near-Death Studies*, found that of 93 veridical perception cases, 92 percent were completely accurate, 6 percent had some errors, and only one case was erroneous.[132] What is observed while the person should be dead is often outside of the unconscious person's line of sight, and may even be of places and people far removed from the location of death. Other cases cite traveling to the home of loved ones, attempting to communicate, and witnessing their activities, even when thousands of miles away.

Pam Reynolds had no oxygen in her brain for over an hour. Could there be another reason she had such elaborate experiences? Perhaps it all stems from aberrant signals in the brain as it shuts down, specifically the temporoparietal junction. This area of the brain integrates information from the visual, auditory, and somatosensory systems (those that involve touch, temperature, pain, motion, and orientation); it is a central area of auditory-verbal hallucinations. Stimulating this spot during surgery can create out-of-body experiences and sensations similar to NDEs.[133] However, perception of the body is again distorted, sensory stimulation is confusing, and the hallucinations involving this area are frightening. With NDEs, which often occur without any stimulation to this part of the brain, sensory information of the body and surroundings are clear, there is heightened lucidity, and the memory is positive and permanent. This biologically based argument also cannot account for veridical experiences, let alone such complex, lucid perception.

A third argument proposes NDEs are due merely to the sudden release of neurotransmitters at death, an evolutionary development designed to cushion our exit. Yet, if this is the final defense mechanism of the body before oblivion, then it serves nothing more than to make us more compliant in the jaws of death. It does not, contrary to the purpose of every other evolutionary development in living organisms, ensure survival. This argument also does not explain veridical phenomena, enhanced memory, profound meaning and peace, and elimination of the fear of death, clarity of perception, or any of the other lasting psychological effects that NDEs have on many survivors.

NDEs are also explained as hallucinations induced by the medications given to comfort patients near the end of life. Ketamine, a drug used in anesthetics, often produces OBEs, but these are frightening, fractured hallucinations, hardly the sophisticated reports of loving spirits and relatives in NDEs.

Another organic argument to account for NDEs is REM intrusion. You've likely experienced this, the state of being caught semi-aware in a dream, either enjoying the experience such as when you're able to fly, or paralyzed by fear when you're trapped in a nightmare. One feels the experience as if it were real; it is auditory and kinetic. REM intrusion can also occur with a lack of oxygen; higher brain areas in the cortex quickly blank out, but the brain stem (since it's more primitive) remains active for several minutes longer. You can experience quite a lot in this state, even though it may only last a short while. In the same way, it is argued, an NDE that seems timeless might occur in the few seconds right before or after the cortex blanks out. Against this we can leverage the same features as before: veridical experience, higher perception, the experience is coherent and meaningful, permanently life-changing, and remembered accurately. Details of a dream during REM intrusion shift and fade with time, unlike NDEs, which remain accurate for years. Furthermore, NDEs may occur while a patient is taking medications that suppress REM, or while in a deep coma, which displays no REM activity.

Finally, the complex experience of NDEs has been attributed to neural fireworks in the dying brain. Such was the perspective of a University of Michigan study, which found that the brain is quite active at the final moments of dying. There is a significant peak in electrical activity moving like a firestorm through the cerebral cortex. It's a last explosion of neural vitality before oblivion.[134] According to the findings, this is more than sufficient to support rich conscious experience, but it's not heaven. It's simply the brain blazing out in a glory very much of this world.

Gaining this insight required execution of a most gruesome nature: decapitation. Researchers lopped the heads off a band of unfortunate rats, monitoring brainwaves in their severed craniums as they died. The "wave of death" lasted about thirty seconds, proportional to the size of a rat's cerebral cortex. This is consistent with what we know from the ICU as we witness people die while under full instrumentation. For years, EEG devices have recorded this death spike, the result of oxygen-starved neurons losing their potassium potential and misfiring. With larger brains, our wave of death lasts approximately three minutes — more than enough time, psychologically speaking, for a complex experience such as an NDE: meeting loved ones, a life review, receiving insight and special knowledge on one's journey, even understanding the mysteries of the universe. Is it a spiritual download or a psychotic delusion? The authors of the study were wisely cautious: "It's one thing to measure brain activity in rats during cardiac arrest, and quite another to relate that to human experience."[135]

Indeed, this represents the fundamental problem with explaining away NDEs as a cascade of electrical chaos in the brain: we are able to observe only the initial metabolic processes of death. We have no way to quantify the subjective experience of the one dying, especially beyond the point of measurable physiological activity. By its nature, death does not lend itself to the scientific method. But while electrical surges in the brain fail to explain NDEs, they may actually indicate the beginning of them. Death is not an event, but a process, and this may be the last measurable moment of that process. Are we witnessing the soul's recognition of heaven just as the last lines are cut to the physical world?

And then there are the many cases of NDEs occurring spontaneously, while in meditation, in heightened emotional states, and in shared experiences. None of these cases involve an EEG surge. Are all these people simply going mad?

PSYCHOLOGICAL EXPLANATIONS

IF THE HEFTY HANDFUL OF ELECTRICAL CONNECTIONS BETWEEN OUR EARS could give rise to such complex experiences as forming identity, making meaning, or falling in love, then it's not such a leap to consider how they may also create mystical experience. Politely, that's called imagination. It's also known as being off your rocker. Could the alternate reality so many touch upon actually be a psychotic episode?

Dr. Bruce Greyson is a leading researcher with the division of perceptual studies at the University of Virginia. He points out, "That assumption can be maintained only by ignoring the profound differences between spiritually transformative experiences and psychotic experiences. These pervasive differences include the context in which the two kinds of experience occur, the content of the experience itself, how the experience is remembered, and how the experience affects the individual. Spiritually transformative experiences, unlike most forms of mental illness, may enhance serenity and sense of purpose and expand the experiencer's perception and appreciation of the world."[136]

Of course, "crazy" is too strong and dismissive a term for the spectrum of conditions we may find ourselves in as we cope with altered perception. Our exploration of these phenomena will be framed in light of positive NDEs, which make up the majority of cases and certainly dominate the bestseller's list.

From the psychological perspective, hallucination is the most common argument used to dismiss NDEs, even though hallucinations are usually illogical, fleeting, bizarre, and/or distorted, whereas NDEs are generally described as more comprehensible and transcendent. They certainly can also be other-worldly, and sometimes frightening. However, according to Kenneth Ring and Bruce Greyson, "People tend to forget their hallucinations, whereas most NDEs remain vivid for decades. Such episodes often lead to profound and permanent transformations in personality, attitudes, beliefs and values — things that are never seen following hallucinations. People looking back on hallucinations typically recognize them as unreal, as fantasies, while people often describe their NDEs as 'more real than real.' Further, people who have experienced both hallucinations and an NDE describe them as being quite different."[137]

Certain mental disorders may be mistaken as explanations for NDEs. Cotard's Syndrome, for instance, is an unsettling state in which individuals believe they are dead when they are not, such as following an accident or war zone trauma. However, memory is blocked in these states, while NDEs heighten memory. Knowledge that one is dead is not unsettling during an NDE, and out-of-body experiences are not present with Cotard's Syndrome.

Perhaps it's depersonalization, a mental discord in which one replaces an unpleasant reality with a fantasy, including observing oneself from outside the body. However, that experience of the body is often distorted, and surroundings can be either blurred and muted or amplified and intense. Memories and perceptions are dulled, marked by little more than emotional numbness. NDEs, on the other hand, are experienced as shifts in consciousness, with increased awareness. When an OBE occurs, perception of the body and its surroundings is accurate with lucid recall of details.

Could the end of life actually be a replay of the beginning? Some have proposed NDEs are simply birth memories, traveling down a tunnel toward a point of light, entering a completely new reality, and being embraced by loving beings. Beyond those surface similarities, the argument quickly falls apart. Birth, for the infant, is traumatic, as contractions force the child out, while the NDE tunnel is often a smooth, swift transition (though some are confusing and stressful). This, again, can be unique to each individual, and many NDEs do not have a tunnel experience at all, they just wake up in another realm.

How about post-traumatic stress disorder (PTSD), the result of exposure to ordeals such as sexual violence, threat of death, or intense suffering? This increasingly common condition debilitates one's functioning and can destroy relationships and careers, leading to complex depression. Symptoms include frightening memories and flashbacks, nightmares, chronic anxiety, sleep disturbances, depersonalization, and a sense of foreboding. "PTSD really can be characterized as a disorder of memory," says McGill University psychologist Alain Brunet, who studies and treats psychological trauma. "It's about what you wish to forget and what you cannot forget."[138] NDEs, however, are mostly pleasant experiences, often in stark contrast to the frightening circumstances from which they arise. They often result in the elimination of the fear of death, not traumatic strain against it.[139,140] Rather than trauma resulting in memory suppression, it is the sheer joy and clarity of NDEs that make them incompatible with this reality, so they are suppressed in order to maintain existential equilibrium. Which brings us to the next argument.

It's simply imagination. Awakening from my own NDE, which was a decidedly spiritual experience, that's the reaction I had as I returned from a love and landscape that left my heart aching. So different was that world from this and so ultimately transformative was my joy that reconciling the two realities was like a deep-sea fish trying to describe a warm, sunlit meadow. So, I gave it a tolerable framework, buried it in my subconscious, and carried on without dealing with its implications. Here's that cognitive dissonance again, the instinctive reaction to hold beliefs and perceptions in harmony when confronted with an alternate reality. This is why it can take decades to integrate the experience. How does one communicate the answers to life's questions when they've been downloaded directly into one's soul? Truths become intuitively known, held beneath language, resonating through experience, art, music, but not the rational mind. And yet, like seeing a mathematical theorem and feeling how its beauty and truth are entwined, the NDE material slowly manifests toward articulation, just as the survivor's life waxes toward remembering what awaits us.

If it wasn't real, if I imagined it, then it should also change over time. That's the way memory works. We are miserable historians, with most people accurately recalling only a small percent of their lives. Decades of research show that memory does not function like a recording. It is constructed and reconstructed throughout time. It functions more like *Wikipedia*, in which others can rewrite it, not just yourself. Memory and imagination are siblings, making false memory a common phenomenon. And, each time a memory is recalled, it becomes vulnerable to mutation through a process called memory reconsolidation.[141] Further, the recollection of whether an experience was good or bad is often determined almost exclusively by its ending. If a pleasant experience ends not so well, the entire event will be remembered as unpleasant. Think of a great movie you saw that ended disappointingly. The whole movie tends to get written off.[142]

From this we can see that memory is terribly inaccurate, undependable, and subjective. Not so with NDEs. In a 2013 study, twenty-one patients who experienced acute brain injury and coma were separated into three groups: those who had an NDE, those who reported memories during coma but without an NDE, and those who reported no memories of their coma. These coma patients were also compared with eighteen healthy control subjects. NDEs were found to have more detail than memories of imagined or real events. They provided more self-referential and emotional information, and had far better clarity than memories during coma.

The study's conclusion: "The subject really perceived these phenomena.

However, since the perceived events did not occur in reality, the perceptions are hallucinatory."[143] If only they had stated instead, "since the perceived events did not occur in *this* reality,…" they could have ended not with the conclusion that it was hallucinatory but that it was revelatory. Nonetheless, the study supports what NDE researchers have found for years: the memory of the event never fades in detail or intensity, even after decades. The emotional texture of such an experience is as fresh as if it just happened. This is consistent with accounts from all the people I have spoken with, and with my own experience as well. Our recollection is charged with the clarity and intensity of the original event. And, as mentioned, these episodes result in permanent changes in people's lives and characters. You cannot return from that country unchanged.

I knew I wanted to see it again. I still do. It is as fresh in my memory as if it happened yesterday. To be honest, so amazing was the experience that I secretly prayed, before every subsequent surgery, that I would have another glimpse. And every time I would wake with disappointment. Why not, I would plead. Why can't I see it again? The response was always the same: silence.

It's fascinating to note the effects survivors experience. Physical alterations can include lower blood pressure, change in sleep patterns, synaesthesia (an involuntary blending of the senses), sensitivity to medications[144] and to electromagnetic emissions (electronic equipment can spontaneously fail).[145] Non-physical changes include stronger positive emotions, increased compassion, alertness, and intuitive awareness. And none of these effects are found in any of the psychological or biological explanations for NDEs. While the biological shifts happen quickly, the rest tend to emerge over time — it's a bumpy road integrating an alternate reality. Usually what follows is a wilderness for a while.

Children seem to have more NDEs than adults when close to death, or perhaps they more easily report it.[146] Interestingly, it appears that far less will have a distressing NDE, possibly because shadow aspects of their subconscious have not yet become dominant. When supported in their experience, children seem to integrate it faster than adults. Many also appear to have heightened compassion, sensitivity to violence, and an increased ability to comprehend abstract concepts.[147] Something very interesting is happening.

While we're pondering the arguments against this life-changing experience being real, it is vital to remember a pivotal point which can make or break the hope NDEs write upon a person's heart: *the cause is not the experience.* Any attempt to explain their story will reduce their story. This individual has just experienced an unparalleled dimension of being. It will become a defining facet of their identity in this world. The best response is an open and compassionate one, whatever you may think of their tale.[148] The significance of this cannot be overstated, even when the details of their story seem to be, for the most critical element of an NDE is actually what happens afterwards — debriefing.

When supported, the event can result in an amazing life of deep compassion, creative expression, meaning, and healing.[149] More often, though, the accounts are met with skepticism, or dismissed as naïve imaginings. No wonder the experience is suppressed, resulting in a unique and private existential tension throughout life. No wonder returnees have higher rates of divorce[150] and depression,[151] and tend to leave career and religion behind (though there is often a marked increase in spirituality).[152] While that may seem odd for someone who's visited heaven, it's in line with the stories of all spiritual pilgrims. Put simply, drawing close to God is going to mess you up. You will not be left comfortable with how things were. Yes, you get to experience a transcendent reality, but returning from this amazing adventure requires your soul to be compacted back into physical form, for you to live once again within the confines and craziness of culture, just after you have tasted an astonishing authenticity and clarity of love. Those are rare and dangerous qualities to live by, yet are the only ones that heal the world. You're back to make a difference, but what is it? If only the acquired wisdom, details, and insights of the experience were not buried in the subconscious, emerging in fragments as the years pass by!

You certainly do not return enlightened. Experiencers stumble, struggle, and strive as much as any other mortal. They have become modern pilgrims who have grazed the edge of immortality. While in ancient times such people would be embraced as shamans or seers, sojourners these days tend to quietly carry their secret, odd ducks in a skeptical world.

HUBRIS AND HOPE

WHILE NDES ARE COMMONLY NOT REVEALED FOR FEAR OF JUDGMENT AND ridicule, there is another understandable reason to keep them private: people may perceive you as boasting. When you think of it, there can be no greater hubris than to say you've been to heaven and chatted with the angels! We see this dynamic not only in modern accounts, but also in one of the most ancient: St. Paul's second letter to the Corinthians, written about twenty years after Jesus died. He relates this experience in a letter called Acts, one of the earliest writings of the Christian scriptures, and then expands upon it in another letter to a church in Corinth. This is a passionate and convoluted document,[153] reprimanding and guiding the church leaders, who had become torn by power plays and sinful behavior. Understanding the context of the account is helpful in exploring the psychological tension of sharing such personal wonders.

Corinth had a young church that was struggling. New, charismatic teachers had caused a split in the community, leading some away from what Paul had taught them about Jesus. With his authority undermined, Paul presented his case with heartfelt passion, defending his credibility against those who boastfully claimed to be "super apostles." This was a time of intense spiritual activity in the church as a whole, with individuals manifesting miraculous powers, prophetic insight, and receiving the spiritual gift of spontaneously speaking in other languages. While Paul had the latter ability, it's important to remember he also had a past that caused many to question his motives. He was not one of the original disciples, and never met Jesus in the flesh. Rather, Paul was a renowned Pharisee, a religious zealot who hunted down and persecuted Christians with a vengeance before his own conversion. That experience resulted in a complete transformation of character, from savagely killing to fearlessly loving. Here's his account:

> While I was on my way and approaching Damascus, about
> noon a great light from heaven suddenly shone about me. I fell
> to the ground and heard a voice saying to me, "Saul, Saul, why
> are you persecuting me?" I answered, "Who are you, Lord?"
> Then he said to me, "I am Jesus of Nazareth, whom you are
> persecuting." Now those who were with me saw the light but
> did not hear the voice of the one who was speaking to me. I
> asked, "What am I to do, Lord?" The Lord said to me, "Get up
> and go to Damascus; there you will be told everything that
> has been assigned to you to do." Since I could not see because
> of the brightness of that light, those who were with me took
> my hand and led me to Damascus.[154]

Even though Paul has a direct encounter with Jesus, it is a mystical one, not physical like the other apostles. How could he further defend his claim as being one of them? In his letter, Paul approaches this from several fronts: his generosity in supporting their community, his history as a Jewish leader, his suffering for the sake of the Gospel, and the details of his conversion. The intensity of his argument is among the most passionate writings in the Bible. Then he reaches a point when he could let his argument stand as is or take it one step further. He chooses to go all out and tell them everything:

> I know a man in Christ who fourteen years ago was caught up
> to the third heaven. Whether it was in the body or out of the
> body I do not know — God knows...this man ... was caught
> up to paradise and heard inexpressible things, things that no
> one is permitted to tell. I will boast about a man like that, but
> I will not boast about myself, except about my weaknesses.
> Even if I should choose to boast, I would not be a fool, because
> I would be speaking the truth. But I refrain, so no one will
> think more of me than is warranted by what I do or say, or
> because of these surpassingly great revelations.[155]

There is so much going on here that parallels NDEs and the effects they have on a person's life. First, notice that Paul refers to the experience happening not to himself, but to another man. This is reinforced in verse 5: "I will boast about a man like that, but I will not boast about myself, except about my weakness." The sentence throws the story into the arena of scholarly debate, with some stating it was a common literary tool to write of yourself in the third person. Given that Paul was responding to the boasting claims made by his rivals of revelations and powers, it makes sense that he state his case without seeming as if he's doing so in the same arrogant spirit as them.

Like those who've had an NDE and encountered celestial beings, Paul claims to have met Jesus:

> Last of all, as to one untimely born, he appeared also to me. For I am the least of the apostles, unfit to be called an apostle, because I persecuted the church of God.[156]

It's difficult for us to comprehend the magnitude of Paul's transformation. Here was a leader among the Pharisees, a group renowned for their strict moral code, revered for their zeal and dedication. They were, in modern terms, self-righteous religionists, very conservative, very strict, and very determined to exterminate the followers of Jesus. And he dove into that slaughter with sadistic glee. What a complete change in character and action! Likewise, after an NDE, people who led disreputable lives of profound cruelty reform their ways, repair their relationships, and strive to embody that indescribable joy and love they encountered on the other side.

As in advanced NDE accounts, Paul goes on to describe understandings gained on the various qualities of energy and consciousness in the heavenly realm — different forms of glory and wonder according to the type of being.[157] He even goes on to describe the unique signatures of glory between stars and planets, indicating a sophisticated spiritual journey with revelations on the nature of creation itself.

Like NDE survivors, Paul looks forward to the day he can return to that loving dimension, but he knows he has a purpose to fulfill here on earth. He relates this in a passionate letter to the Philippians. It is a document infused with spiritual conviction:

> For to me, to live is Christ and to die is gain. If I am to go on living in the body, this will mean fruitful labor for me. Yet what shall I choose? I do not know! I am torn between the two: I desire to depart and be with Christ, which is better by far; but it is more necessary for you that I remain in the body.[158]

Paul now had something to stand for that was bigger than himself. It called him to make a difference in the world, to open to other's suffering, to practice profound compassion, to win them to love. Yet, loving so courageously in such a brutal culture placed him in great danger and led him down a path that included imprisonment, torture, starvation, shipwrecks, poverty, ridicule, and, ultimately, execution. Few people are as qualified as Paul to speak of their suffering as being all for the sake and glory of God.

Finally, the most significant impact NDEs have on survivors, one which Paul's narrative illustrates, is the realization that love is so much more than an emotion — it is the ground of reality itself, the highest form of evolutionary consciousness, the very imprint of the Divine within us.

LOVE IS THE BOTTOM LINE

I WAS PRIVILEGED TO HEAR A BEAUTIFUL EXAMPLE OF THAT POWER AND love. Olaf and Ruth were an elderly couple in my first parish. Now in their nineties, they had lived off the land since escaping Norway during the Nazi occupation, settling in the harsh Saskatchewan prairie and building a beautiful, modest life. This first visit from the new young pastor was a great pleasure for them and an honor for me. I felt excited and grateful as we sat to share a simple snack and the stories of life. Somehow the tales turned to the topic of Olaf's NDE, an incident which renewed his faith and changed his life.

"I didn't want to come back. I love you with all my heart, but I just didn't want to come back." Olaf was holding Ruth's hands, tears streaming down his cheeks while the memory of the land he had seen filled him as if he had been there just yesterday. Except, this was thirty years later. I sat in their kitchen with my cookies and tea, wide-eyed with curiosity.

"I was in the bathroom and slipped in the tub. There I was, suddenly outside of my body. I could see myself, lying there with a bloody head, but I wasn't afraid. Then I saw this light and was suddenly in a place...so beautiful, so beautiful ..." Ruth squeezed his hand.

Then, he looked at me, and a floodgate opened. "All the waste! All the waste and killing and foolishness! If we'd only realize! We hurt each other when there could be so much love!" He went on to express his grief, pain, and anger that the world continued to career down a path of destruction when just on the other side of the veil lay a foundation of love and connection so breathtaking that it left him weeping at the table. "I didn't want to come back here." He looked to his wife. "But I heard you calling."

"That's right!" she said, looking at me. "I came in the bathroom and there he was. I was so afraid! I said, "Olaf! Olaf!"

"Yes," he said. "I heard you but I didn't want to come back."

"He never listens to me!" she said, tapping his hand. We laughed.

I looked at his eyes, his quivering hands. "You feel it so vividly."

"It was a long time ago. But I know it. I'll never forget." He patted his wife's hand, touched her cheek. "We don't have to be afraid."

We're evolving into love itself. Olaf knew that to the bone and beyond. So did Paul. He spelled this out in one of the most well-known passages from the Bible. Here, Paul drops the mic on those who would boast of their spiritual powers. He lays down the line on love, with a conviction that he has seen that realm, and it is our home:

> If I speak in the tongues of mortals and of angels, but do not have love, I am a noisy gong or a clanging cymbal. And if I have prophetic powers, and understand all mysteries and all knowledge, and if I have all faith, so as to remove mountains, but do not have love, I am nothing. If I give away all my

possessions, and if I hand over my body so that I may boast, but do not have love, I gain nothing.

Love is patient; love is kind; love is not envious or boastful or arrogant or rude. It does not insist on its own way; it is not irritable or resentful; it does not rejoice in wrongdoing, but rejoices in the truth. It bears all things, believes all things, hopes all things, endures all things.

Love never ends. But as for prophecies, they will come to an end; as for tongues, they will cease; as for knowledge, it will come to an end. For we know only in part, and we prophesy only in part; but when the complete comes, the partial will come to an end. When I was a child, I spoke like a child, I thought like a child, I reasoned like a child; when I became an adult, I put an end to childish ways. For now we see in a mirror, dimly, but then we will see face to face. Now I know only in part; then I will know fully, even as I have been fully known. And now faith, hope, and love abide, these three; and the greatest of these is love.[159]

St. Paul and Olaf, along with millions of others, are saying the clarity experienced when their consciousness shifted to the spiritual realm was a wild wake-up to wonder. That day will come for everyone. We will understand the meaning of life as clearly as God understands us. Even more, Paul says, as important as faith and hope are, they will fall away. They are not eternal; they are not the most important qualities of spirit. They, ultimately, won't get you connected to God like love will. So many facing cancer have told me they've lost their faith or they don't know what to believe. So many have said they've lost hope, they can't reach for a future any longer. They feel they are in the darkest moments of life, yet if there is love, then the most important work of the soul is already being done. That work, of course, is also the hardest.

JOE

I MET JOE AT AN ESPECIALLY DARK TIME IN HIS LIFE. STAFF HAD ASKED me to assess him for distress and risk of suicide as he dealt with aggressive throat cancer; he had only a few months to live. At first he seemed calm and collected, but this was, in fact, disengagement. He struggled with depression, and during a particularly low point three years ago, he had attempted suicide by overdosing. A recluse most of his life, his manner now was aloof; he made little eye contact, and was unusually deferential. Something about him, though, made me think another suicide attempt was unlikely.

I went through the standard assessment: Joe was sleeping well; his appetite was normal, considering the condition of his throat and ability to swallow. He had endured difficult surgery to the throat and heavy radiation, which had left his face and neck burned and scarred, but these procedures were to improve swallowing, breathing, and basic quality of life. His treatment was going to result in more physical suffering. There was a possibility he would have to use tube feeding, in addition to disfigurement and the destruction of his saliva glands. It was going to be a rough road.

He had a girlfriend (his first), a kind and compassionate woman who, to his frustration, kept pushing him to connect more with his family, communicate openly with her, and consider a life broader than sitting in his apartment alone with his dog. This, to him, was the main stress in his life. He didn't like the attention, he generally felt awkward with people, as if he was under constant scrutiny and judgment. We discussed where this might have originated. The family history began to unfold.

His father had abused Joe as a child, both verbally and sexually. He had been taunted and bullied in school. He had been unable to form significant and lasting relationships. The foundational message had formed: I am unlovable. I am worthless. I am nothing. For years, this critical voice, this central pain circulated within Joe. It was a message he believed, which led to depression, withdrawal, and escape from this world.

Passive thoughts of suicide are common among cancer patients.[160] The risk of actual suicide becomes significant if there have been attempts in the past, especially among men, and this is even higher with oral cancer. While healthcare professionals are bound to report any suicidal ideation and have the patient psychiatrically assessed, suicide was decriminalized in Canada in 1972. Compassion, genuine care, and decisive insight are needed to assess and support those at risk, for beneath the threat lies profound pain and isolation, so great that death feels like the only escape. For Joe, this was a legitimate concern.

"Do you feel like escaping again?" I asked. "Given the treatment and cancer, do you feel suicide would be better?"

"No", said Joe. "I don't think about that. I know that wouldn't work."

A clue. Why the confidence behind that statement?

"Joe, do you remember anything from when you tried suicide?"

A pause. I suspected he had a near-death experience and hadn't told anyone. Would he tell me?

"There were two doors. I was dead and went through this tunnel, which ended at two doors. I wanted to open the one with the light behind it, but I couldn't. It was locked. And then I heard a voice say, 'You can't come. It's not your time, you have to go back.' I didn't want to open the other door, 'cause I knew it would lead back here. But there was nowhere else to go. I knew from the voice there was no other choice."

"Why do you think you were sent back? Why couldn't you go further?"

"I don't know. I don't know. But when I came back here, I didn't feel judged, or bad. I hadn't been rejected. I just knew it wasn't my time. There was more for me to do."

Silence.

"Have you told anyone else about this experience?"

"No. You're the only one."

This was another case of a person who held the experience within his heart, fearing ridicule, questioning if it was real at all. For such a long time, these individuals think they're alone and that no one could ever understand. It's critical to be open and accepting of near-death accounts when a person first shares their story, even if it occurred years before. A compassionate and curious stance can open the survivor's memory and release a floodgate of emotional energy long compartmentalized in the effort to maintain balance in the face of touching a completely different reality. This is all the more true when the account is a result of suicide, an experience burdened with guilt, shame, regret, and longing.

While Christianity has taught that suicide results in eternal separation from God because it is the rejection of God's greatest gift — life — NDE accounts paint a more complex story. Research reveals no correlation between suicide and negative NDEs. Sometimes those who attempt suicide are shown through a life review why their emotional pain was so great. The compassion of this helps to heal that profound wound of the soul. When they are sent back, most have no desire to take their life again.[161] They instead want to live their life well.

While it would be comforting to think that all who return have a new-found compassion for themselves and a clearer insight into the path which led them to such a dark place, most actually continue to stumble along life's way. How wonderful if, through an NDE, forgiveness and release of the pain carried through the years would be automatic.

"Well, you're not alone," I said. "Millions of people have these experiences, and I hear at least one every month. You are among a sea of humanity that has glimpsed a wider shore and come back to tell us about it. You discovered that you don't fall off the edge of the earth when you reach the end." His eyes were fixed on me, his expression hopeful and cautious. I continued.

"There are many accounts of suicide attempts, and your story is not unlike theirs. Some have an out-of-body experience, travel through a tunnel, encounter a loving powerful being but also a barrier, and are told to come back. They may have a life review, in which they come to understand how the pain built in their soul finally resulted in attempting suicide. But this is presented with absolute compassion. On returning, they struggle to love, to matter, to find that purpose. This is clear for some, difficult for others. So, Joe, it makes me wonder … what's your homework? Why were you sent back?"

He stared blankly past my shoulder, lost in the memory of his experience, desperately reaching for an answer that had eluded him for years. "I don't know. I don't know." His eyes moved slightly to gaze back into mine, hoping for an answer, and I had the audacity to give it to him, because it was staring me in the face. It was love. It always is.

"Joe, which relationships give you the most joy? With whom are you happiest?"

No hesitation in his answer: "My dog. I just love being with my dog. I prefer him to people, you know. He just makes me so happy."

This was no surprise. Gilda Radner once described dogs as "the role model for being alive." Joe found the safest love in the one creature that gives it unconditionally, and that was the limit of his comfort zone. He would not allow his mother's love in; her inaction made her an accomplice in his father's abuse. He would not let his girlfriend in; she was pushing him back into the embrace of the person who should have protected him. Her love itself felt risky: how could he open his heart when it was dominated by his original injury? So, in the cycle of failed friendships and fractured intimacy, his ability to love himself had died. He was a stranger to his own heart, unaware of his dignity or his power.

"That makes so much sense, Joe. Your dog provides you with the best love we can learn from. But you're meant not just to be loved by him but also to love others with a heart that is so grounded that it is not defined by how others have hurt you or failed you. You're meant to love with a heart that can be vulnerable and strong, open and invincible. That's God's heart, God's love. That's who you met at those doors, and you couldn't go in because you can't, as yet, exist there. It's too pure in love. You've got some evolving to do before you can handle that. So, you were sent back to practice, to grow in love, to grow into what you are meant to be so you can continue over there."

Joe sat silently receiving my words, shifting with the implications. If this was what he was supposed to do, he didn't like it. It meant letting those who loved him in to his pain. It meant opening up. It meant breaking the old patterns. Life was going to get very uncomfortable.

"The stakes couldn't be higher," I continued. "This is not only for your sake, but also for the sake of your family. This is about their healing, their evolution in love as well as yours. And, you have a deadline, literally. What are you going to do?"

"What am I going to do? I don't know."

"Why don't you start by talking with your girlfriend about what happened. Does she know?"

"No."

"Hmm. Sounds like you've got an interesting conversation ahead of you."

Joe left that day equipped with a new understanding: his experience wasn't a hallucination, and the message from the doorway was a mystery he was meant to solve. These ideas brought him comfort and curiosity, but the notion that he had to open up to those who loved him, that he had to let them in to the pain he held since childhood — that was terrifying. It triggered the violent and repressed memory of abuse, a profound truth that needed a voice. It would take counseling and support, but he did not have that much time left. I could only hope that the work he began here would be completed on the other side of that doorway.

I never saw Joe again, but was grateful to hear months later that he eventually shared his story and moved in with his girlfriend. With his mother, she cared for him until his peaceful death. Joe had engaged with the most courageous act of self-compassion, to no longer plunge the blade of unlovability into his own heart. He stopped hiding from love. He learned to trust it, and I'm confident that he was eventually transformed by it.

CHAPTER 18

REDEEMING ATONEMENT

To experience what isn't, love what is.

— ERIC MICHA'EL LEVENTHAL

STEVEN SITS ON THE EDGE OF THE BED, THE WARM MORNING SUN slowly pushing back the shadow on his face. He leans back from its radiance as he speaks. "I just can't believe it. The doc was in here talking about the odds. She actually said they don't know what to do. They don't know …" He shakes his head.

He is only thirty-eight. Father of a beautiful four-year-old son, the treasure of his heart, loving husband to a wonderful wife who adores him, son of proud parents who could not ask for a better man to continue their legacy. Except that he likely will not. His stem cell transplant has bought him only five months, despite the close bond he has with his brother, who donated the elixir they prayed would save his life. His body, no longer toned and muscular despite efforts at rebuilding, is now a shade darker. The transplant has given him his brother's hair, which covers him like a furry mat. He removes his sock to show me the top of his foot.

"Look at me. I'm an ape now!" We both laugh. "At least it covers the rash." That developed a few nights before. Within a couple of hours, uneven red splotches had spread head to toe. "The docs couldn't decide if it was graft vs. host or the leukemia. One even thinks the cancer is in my spine. Cancer in my spine ..." Steven's eyes are watering in the light. He shifts his position to the shadow at the end of the bed, away from the brilliance. "My mouth has turned white, and the left side of my body has lost all muscle tone." He flexes a flaccid bicep. "What the hell is happening? This was supposed to work. Now I don't know if I'll make it to Christmas."

We talk. Well, he talks; I listen. He talks about what he'd rather be doing than sitting here in the hospital. For years, he's been restoring two Chevy Camaros, showing his son the tools, mentoring his legacy, his pride and joy. If only he could be repaired as easily. He feels helplessness, like a pincushion, relying on the medicine and expertise of team members who confess they are at a loss. Now consulting with centers across North America, they are searching for answers, options, anything.

"I lie here waiting. At the end of my life, I should be doing more than waiting." We talk about his son. We look at family pictures. We sit with the tears as the sunlight edges closer.

Later in the day I'm wrapping up emails when a knock comes at the door. I turn to see the wheelchair. It's John, Steven's father, a grizzly bear of a man more accustomed to his garage and mechanic's tools than the sterile environment of a cancer floor.

"Can I chat with ya for a minute?"

"Sure!" I reply. "Be happy to."

He rolls in, not making eye contact. Oil-stained hands grip the armrests as he speaks. "You gotta do something to lift Steven's spirits." His eyes are already moist. "He's been down ever since they said it could be in his spine. He doesn't sleep. He just looks at the pictures of Cody. That boy is why he's fighting. He can't give up. But he just lies there, quiet." John pauses, wipes his eyes, looks at me. "They don't know what to do. I don't know what to do."

Don't speak. Don't say anything. Hold his eyes, hold his pain. He begins to weep. "I'm really scared."

We discuss all Steven has been through. The transplant had actually gone smoothly. No medications were needed for mouth sores, time in the hospital was brief, strength steadily returned. It seemed he was in the clear until the fatigue came, then the cough and nerve pain. That's when he took some Advil so he could get a good night's sleep, but it also masked a fever that was brewing, an indication something bigger was going on. It could have been graft vs. host disease — the most common complication after a stem cell transplant — or worse.

That's precisely what the tests revealed. The cancer had returned, and was spreading quickly. If he hadn't taken the Advil, the fever would have been caught peaking over 38˚C three weeks earlier, and he automatically would have been admitted. Perhaps it didn't matter in the end. If it was graft vs. host, he would have ended up in the hospital anyway for symptom management with specialized medications not available at a pharmacy. And the reality was, we had no more cards up our sleeves. The transplant had failed. It gave him only five months. Another transplant would surely kill him because the chemotherapy needed to hit his disease as hard as possible would be more than his weakened body could tolerate.

The team did decide to try a low-dose, long-term chemo procedure, but it was a shot in the dark. Truth was, until they could find an alternative to the standard of care used worldwide, the best that could be done was to manage his symptoms. It left him feeling powerless. It left him to do the preparatory work of grief when all he wanted was hope.

That hope came, but not to Steven, and not as expected. It came to his father. And it scared the life out of him.

"You gotta tell me if I'm crazy," John said, hands now trembling. "Something happened last night. I don't know if it was real or a dream. I don't know what is was."

I knew he was about to share something amazing. I silently prayed for the wisdom to help him understand its significance.

"I was sleeping. And then I felt this presence, opened my eyes … I think I opened my eyes … and they were standing there, at the foot of the bed: my mother, Cheryl's mother, and her aunt with her. Cheryl didn't wake up, she didn't know."

He was looking at me to see a reaction, a confirmation, an expression that would tell him it's safe to continue the tale. This is a critical stage, at the beginning, when words first tumble out. You wonder if the other will accept your story, or if they will just be kind, or worse, polite. I leaned forward, nodding, my eyes a little wider. John continued.

"My mom died years ago, Cheryl's mom and aunt a few years after that. I'm not a religious man. I left the church after Mom died, and I don't care to go back with what happened to Steven. It's not like I gave up on God. I just couldn't believe how cold they were, how they didn't care. I've got no use for that." His eyes held anger and grief, loneliness and love for his son. He was crying as he gently rocked back and forth in the chair. "But there they were, standing and smiling at me, and Mom said, 'We're right here with you. He won't be alone.' Cheryl's mom said, 'We'll be with Steven through all of this.' Her sister was nodding and said, 'Don't worry,' like she always did when things got bad."

"How did you feel as this was happening?" I asked.

"Scared out of my mind!" John exclaimed. "Didn't know what to do! Couldn't move, couldn't even speak. Closed my eyes. I think I turned to Cheryl, then looked back. They were gone. Was I sleeping? I don't remember. Didn't tell her until the morning. Wasn't going to say anything, but I couldn't shake it. Am I crazy?"

It was a delicate gift to affirm his experience. I talked about the soul, the evidence that it continues after death, the privilege I have to frequently hear a story from someone who's glimpsed the other side and come back. I shared how common visitations from deceased relatives are, how maddening they can be when the message remains ambiguous. What a frustration, to receive communication from the beyond and not clearly understand its meaning! Will Steven live or die? That was the bottom line. To me it seemed clear: Steven would die, but spiritual love and strength would sustain him and his family. He would not pass from this world unsupported, and his parents would see him on the other side when their day came. How do you say that when the person in front of you is filled with grief and apprehension, trembling on the edge of admission for fear that saying the words will make it so?

"You can trust this vision," I told him. "It was real. That also means they came to support you, because things are going to get harder. What do you want to do with that information?" I wondered if he would tell Steven.

"It was real?"

"Yes." The shock of that was more than enough to deal with at the moment. Where he would go with that was for him to think about for a while.

"Jesus!" was all he said. I smiled.

"Well, not Jesus, but some of his new friends." The correction was as much to change that expression as to affirm the experience.

By then it was late in the day. Even standing at the edge of heaven, the affairs of Earth continue, and I had to pick my daughter up from school. Perhaps it was best to let John sleep on this, come back to it another time. He would need to contemplate, to integrate, and to listen for the strength this other-worldly visit offered.

"I know you're not a religious man, John, but I'd like to say a prayer with you."

"Yes, yes!" He seems animated and relieved. I held his hands. "Gracious God, thank you. Thank you for this message of love and support. May your spirit consecrate Steven with that same hope — that he is not alone. Whatever may come, you are with him. You are with his family. In that love, may they feel surprisingly safe. May you bless them and keep them. May your face shine upon them and be gracious to them. May you look upon them with favor, and give them peace. Amen."

Down the hall, Steven slept. The sunlight had come and gone, the shadows driven away had returned to enfold him. That was what he needed for now. That's what they all needed, but I knew it would not be long before he would feel light upon his face again. When that happened, there would be no need to shrink back from its brilliance.

ATONEMENT

"IF YOU TALK TO GOD, YOU ARE PRAYING; IF GOD TALKS TO YOU, YOU HAVE schizophrenia. If the dead talk to you, you are a spiritualist; if you talk to the dead, you are a schizophrenic."[162] This insight from psychiatrist Thomas Szasz summarizes the silence of so many that have a near-death experience or a bedside visit from deceased loved ones. They withhold these mystical encounters for fear of being labeled as mentally ill. Speaking up can result in being dismissed by loved ones, excommunicated from your faith community, or, not so long ago, thrown in an asylum. No wonder John was rattled.

Wouldn't it be wonderful if the organization that should be an expert in this area — the church — fully supported people by helping them integrate the experience? Here we have the most profound opportunity to deepen one's faith, but too often the Christian community is silent on the subject or condemns it as occult. There is a large portion of the church that supports spiritually transformative experiences, even more so as stories flood our culture through books, blogs, and films. But knowledge of the cross-cultural, historical, and psychodynamic elements of NDEs is still sadly lacking among clergy. My hope, of course, is that this book will help address that gap.

Conservative Christian groups commonly reject NDEs, even though there are many accounts of born-again Christians experiencing exactly what the Bible, and their church, say they should experience at death: dwelling in paradise, meeting angels and Jesus, seeing the city of God. The rejection comes from doctrinal tension around two core issues. First, NDEs include non-Christians being accepted into heaven, which is incompatible with an interpretation of scripture that understands salvation as exclusive to those who have accepted Christ as their savior through baptism or a personal, heartfelt prayer. Second, NDE accounts often include the idea of reincarnation, which stands at odds with the doctrine of atonement: that Jesus died for our sins, the core of the Christian faith. Does one get to heaven because of the saving act of Christ's death and resurrection or through a series of incarnations that eventually purify the soul?

I'd like to wrestle with these issues in the hope of encouraging reflective consideration that the afterlife is more complex than we realize, and the Christian faith is as much an expression of society as it is a witness to the eternal truths of God made visible through Christ.

Faith, like all aspects of humanity, is in evolution. We must outgrow any concepts of God that reflect more our cultural psychology than Divine Love, which sustains the universe in every moment. While some who read this might be active in a church and familiar with many of the terms, I also want to speak to the growing numbers who have had no exposure to religious language and the loaded symbology of the ancient stories. And, if you will indulge me for this chapter, I need to speak as a member of the clergy as I explore why you don't need to be a Christian to go to heaven.

The crux of my perspective is summed up in the teaching of Jesus to a lawyer, recorded in Luke 10:25–28.

> Just then a lawyer stood up to test Jesus. "Teacher," he said, "what must I do to inherit eternal life?" He said to him, "What is written in the law? What do you read there?" He answered, "You shall love the Lord your God with all your heart, and with all your soul, and with all your strength, and with all your mind; and your neighbor as yourself." And he said to him, "You have given the right answer; do this, and you will live."

Interestingly, the story goes on with the lawyer asking, "But who is my neighbor?" Turns out (like most of us) he was fine loving people that he was comfortable with. So, Jesus describes how this love is supposed to push us out of our comfort zone, extend openly and completely to others, especially those who society rejects. He does this through what has become one of the most quoted stories of unconditional love, the tale of the Good Samaritan, in which a Levite (one with sacred duties in the temple), a priest, and a Samaritan (who were despised by the Israelites) walk by a man beaten and left for dead. Only the Samaritan helps him. At the end of the tale, Jesus asks the lawyer at Luke 10:36–37,

> "Which of these three, do you think, was a neighbor to the man who fell into the hands of the robbers?" He said, "The

one who showed him mercy." Jesus said to him, "Go and do likewise."

We are challenged to love beyond the labels of who deserves it, who is like us, who matters. We are challenged to ultimately identify ourselves and everyone else as children of God, expressions of the One Consciousness. We do this by allowing only love to be the top priority in life.

During the life review in an NDE, these priorities are revealed. You are shown how you have either advanced the cause of love, or held it back. This is not romantic love (*eros*) or love between friends (*phileo*), but an unconditional love (*agape*), a kind of love that emanates from the very essence and nature of the Divine. Love is what God is, not just something God does. There is no better description of God than this simple word, which we take for granted, yet is the fullness of our hope and destiny. God is described this way in 1 John 4:7–12:

> Dear friends, let us love one another, for love comes from God. Everyone who loves has been born of God and knows God. Whoever does not love does not know God, because God is love. This is how God showed his love among us: He sent his one and only Son into the world that we might live through him. This is love: not that we loved God, but that he loved us and sent his Son as an atoning sacrifice for our sins. Dear friends, since God so loved us, we also ought to love one another. No one has ever seen God; but if we love one another, God lives in us and his love is made complete in us.

All you need is love, as the song goes, and all of us love imperfectly. Thankfully, it is our ability, not our consistency, to love that enables God to meet us more than halfway. No better expression of this is found than in the life, death, and resurrection of Jesus. Here is God going all the way, compassion incarnate, and willing to endure the worst of humanity without wavering in love. After all, St. John did say "This is love: not that we loved God, but that he loved us." Jesus identified fully with God. He and God are one. God is love. Jesus is Love. The Spirit is Love. And in a critical prayer Jesus said just before he was arrested, he asked God that we would be one with him, just as he is one with God, that we would not just feel love, but *be* love as well. When a person experiences this, their love becomes praise as it flows in response to who God is. The more we love, the more we come to know this: that we are to be one with God. Jesus came to remind us of that.

If you are a Christian and troubled by my concept of salvation through love, you may wonder, what of the crucifixion? What of the passage above mentioning atonement through Christ? As a Christian minister, it's important I explore that, and I want to do so in such a way that those who have rejected the notion that Christ died for our sins (sacrificial atonement) can still come to know Him as the fullest expression of God made human, an individual unique in His ability to know Himself as fully connected to His source.

Atonement, at-one-ment, is fundamentally about solidarity, and here is where the crucifixion can make sense for any age. Think of the pains in your life, the wounds you wear from the wreckage of the past, the scars you endure from your own choices, as well as those of others. Perhaps you messed up; perhaps someone messed you up. We tend to carry these broken parts of ourselves secretly, quietly. We push them away or push them down — anything but deal with them. Deep in our hearts is the hope that we can finally be whole, but most of us end up just trying to cope. This is especially true if you have cancer. Yet, we cannot be healed if we deny the depth of our pain. What we're looking for is salvation, as that literally means to be made whole. What to do?

Have you ever noticed what it's like to witness someone take their pain and name it, speak it, share the story, and then state their strength? "I survived. This is what happened to me, this is what I did, and I am aware of it. I survived it. Now, I will do something with it. It did not, it cannot, destroy me, and I will not be defined by it. I have become something greater. And you can, too."

You hear it at any 12-step meeting. "Hi, I'm ____, and I'm an alcoholic." "Hi, I'm ____, and I'm an addict." "I'm a survivor of abuse." They do it by speaking to your hidden pain and saying, "Me too." These people give strength through suffering, hope through endurance, they give tomorrows through being real with today.

That's solidarity, and that's the heart of the incarnation, the crucifixion, and the resurrection. In these three acts, God says, Me too. I know love and friendship and grief. I know pain, rejection, and betrayal. I know death. I have traveled the human journey. I know your story. I understand.

Even more, in Jesus God shows us what we are to be, that death isn't the end of the story, that love is stronger than any mess, any atrocity, any disease. That's the move from God's side. What of our move? Salvation must be more than "whoever lives lovingly goes to heaven." That's too simple. It must be "whoever evolves in love resonates with God, and has the Spirit within them." This is how we are made "a new creation." It is about so much more than being good or nice or moral. This is about the energetic essence of one's being shifting, as a step in evolution, into a new kind of being, a new species if you will.[163] That's the atonement.[164]

Unfortunately, the ancient concept that God demands a blood sacrifice persists in the church. The church through the ages has used this along with a good measure of guilt to maintain political control. Yet the reality of humanity's depravity, and the power of guilt as a motivator for change, need not be co-opted by that agenda. That's what spurred the Protestant reformation, begun by Martin Luther in 1517. His effort was to reform the image of a judging God, who still demanded sacrifice, to an all-loving God, who claims us as his own even before we turn to Him.

God doesn't care so much *who* we love; God cares *that* we love. And what God seems to care about most is that those who love become love itself, just as God is. According to 1 John 4:7, "Everyone who loves has been born of God and knows God." This must be true across cultures and time, faiths and traditions, language and age, for those who lived before Jesus and those after. Cancer can accelerate this growth, slapping us with a reality check and a literal deadline to get serious about love. This is a goal that goes far beyond surviving. It is the purpose of life: to attain the highest level of consciousness through love, a process that cannot be completed here, but continues toward perfection in the life to come.

I have witnessed many brave the task of loving fiercely in the face of death, without wavering. These have been the most beautiful and heartbreaking moments of my ministry.

Until Death Do Us Part

HER TEARS WERE THE ANOINTING. AS SHE LAY WITH HER HEAD ON HIS quiet chest, the sobs rising from deep within her, I knew the blessing of her love was more powerful than any holy oil I could offer, which is why the real moment of consecration came not through any ritual of last rites, but in the giving and receiving of vows. I had been called to the ICU to marry them.

Richard had been a strong man in his early thirties, soon-to-be manager of his own home improvement store, a dream on the edge of realization. He had worked with his father all his life, learning the details of business and following a line of succession that went back three generations. His fiancée, Karen, seemed like heaven's gift, complementing his business skills with her warmth for people and her creativity. Together, they planned the new store: location and layout, suppliers and product. Together, they broke the ground for construction and were about to cut the ribbon for the grand opening. But he felt increasingly tired, wasn't able to concentrate, and then, one morning, noticed the jaundice in his eyes. Kidney cancer strikes suddenly. Because of its rapid growth, five-year survival is very low, around 8 percent if not caught at the earliest stage. Richard and Karen barely had eight weeks between diagnosis and the ICU.

I had seen him in dialysis the week before. He didn't say much. Already frail, his skin took on the deep orange indicating liver failure. But what he did say was loud and clear: he wanted to get well enough to marry Karen. That was the priority. The store could wait, their new home could wait, but this, his heart's desire, could not.

I suggested a bedside ceremony. Not the dream they were hoping for, but certainly a step toward it. They could have a big celebration later. (Though I knew he would die, one never takes a patient's hope away, for even that dream can give vitality to life in the present moment.) Richard liked the idea, but wanted to see how he felt on the weekend before proceeding. He never got the chance. The next morning, everything started to fail. He was rushed downstairs, where Karen echoed his words in the ICU.

"We want to get married. It's all he was fighting for. It's all that matters now. I can't stand to lose him without becoming his wife."

Richard was dying. Sedated and intubated, the machines had been keeping him alive through the night. There was no hope left, except the one that cried from her heart. "I know it would be symbolic, I know he can't respond, but it's what he was hanging on for." Family quietly wept as they stood by the bed: his parents, his uncle, her mother. They all nodded quietly.

To pledge one's love to another, to promise to be faithful until death, is the commitment to honor the light in the other at all times, even when they do not honor it in themselves. Through the commitment of love and the eyes of the heart, we obtain the highest wisdom possible that empowers us to never give up on our connection to each other. This is the awareness that love is so much more than an emotion — an interconnection so deep that, ultimately, we are one. There was no doubt that this couple was already husband and wife in that respect. They simply needed someone to proclaim it.

"It would be a privilege," I said. Everyone drew close as she took his hand in hers, and we closed ours eyes in prayer. The sound of the monitors seemed to recede as we connected to the heart of life. "Gracious God, we gather with hearts filled with grief and love, pain and sorrow. This is so sad. This is so sad. What can we do?" My words were silenced at that point by welling empathy, tears caught on the edge of expression. Yet, sadness is a positive emotion, one that draws us closer to others through shared vulnerability. Sadness increases connection, deepening our humanity. (Depression is the opposite, isolating us, cutting off the vital connections of belonging and understanding.) This actually makes sadness the most powerful opportunity for love to forge the deepest bonds. We spend so much energy avoiding that authenticity, and thus avoiding ourselves.

Held in that moment of silence, I breathed into the sadness and waited for the words to continue.… "What can we do but love? May your love be here, gracious God, in the hearts of Karen and Richard as they pledge to be husband and wife. May you bless them, may their love be stronger than death, forever joining them in the journey that awaits Richard and in the years that unfold for Karen. Consecrate them in your purpose and receive their heart's desire as we thank you for the gift, which makes all things possible, love itself."

He didn't need to be able to speak. I bent low and quietly asked the question that is so traditionally said under vaulted church spires, not beneath respiration monitors and the tangle of tubes and blood lines. "Richard, do you take Karen to be your wife, to have and to hold, for richer, for poorer, in sickness and in health, and forsaking all others, to be faithful to her until death parts you?" (Never do those words strike so powerfully as when said in a hospital.) "Karen, do you take Richard to be your husband, to have and to hold, for richer, for poorer, in sickness and in health, and forsaking all others, to be faithful to him until death parts you?"

"I do," she whispered through her tears.

"Having declared your intention, repeat after me your vow to become husband and wife." The vows were said, Karen to Richard with her head on his chest, Richard to Karen from the beating of his heart. And then things got awkward. A kiss seals the promise, but Karen could not reach his lips — the bed was raised too high! She quickly grabbed a chair and climbed to her love, reached over to embrace him, and astonishingly beamed as she gently kissed his fading face over and over again.

"I love you, I love you." Tears of anointing, breath of life fading, silence of God as Richard's consciousness slipped from her embrace into the arms of the angels.

KAREN AND RICHARD WERE UNITED IN THE SPIRIT OF MARRIAGE LONG before our ceremony in the ICU. Since, through love, consciousness survives death, Karen fully expected Richard to be linked to her for the rest of her life, perhaps even to give her a sign. Despite how common this is throughout the world, people still wonder if they're imagining things, and imagination makes it much more unsettling than it needs to be.

Mother and daughter sat in my office with excitement and trepidation. They had come to ask questions of consciousness, how the soul can continue after death, and most importantly, if the deceased could ever communicate back. As much as they wanted to know Tammy was okay, they weren't sure they could handle it if she somehow let them know. Tammy had died three months earlier, a beautifully peaceful transition through which her mom and sister were forever changed.

"It was remarkable how she didn't suffer, despite the pain. She was filled with gratitude for everyone. So beautiful." Her sister, Sandra, was teary as she recalled the moment. "It was late, the same day you prayed with her, but late in the evening. Her eyes had been closed for most of the day, but then they opened and she looked up to the corner of the room, and said, "Oh, hi!" We knew she was looking at someone, and then she smiled ..." Sandra paused as she felt the moment again. "She paused, and said 'home.' Home. The way she looked ... and then closed her eyes, and that was it. Amazing."

"I'm so glad you were there," I said. "That's the sacred moment that will leave an indelible mark of hope on you. Who do you think greeted her?"

"It must have been her grandmother and cousin," Tammy's mom said. "They were so close. It really was amazing. But we were wondering ... during your prayer, you encouraged her to watch over her kids, to let us know she was okay, but not to 'freak us out.' It made us laugh at the time ..."

"Has something happened?" I asked. "Has Tammy given you a signal that scared you?"

"Yes!" Sandra blurted out. "I'm not sure I want her to do that. I've even been scared to go to sleep, like she might appear in my bedroom. And then, one night, I heard on the baby monitor one of my son's toys just start up on its own. I rushed in there and checked it … it couldn't have done that by itself. Was it her?"

I recalled stories from other family members over the years of similar incidents. These fears are ancient, a tug of war between missing the departed and dreading if their apparition should ever haunt you. Throughout history, entire spiritual systems have developed around ancestral contact, but these have been mediated by the shaman, the one gifted with the ability others dread.

We discussed mediumship as seen on television and stage shows, and its presence in the Bible. In 1 Samuel 28:7–20 we hear the desperation of King Saul. He has ruined his relationship with God, and now faces David, who will be king, in battle. In desperation he goes to the witch of Endor and asks her to summon the spirit of Samuel, a great prophet, for advice on how to defeat David and restore his own glory. The apparition appears, but only to tell Saul that he will die in battle.

Sandra and her mom had sought no medium to assist them. In fact, they were hesitant to have the encounter at all. But if it happened in ancient times, if the celebrity mediums of our day are authentic, what could they do to discern Tammy's spirit if she should try to contact them?

"Focus on the love," I advised them. "If you're lying in bed dreading the thought of her appearing, you're being driven by your fear. Fear is of the ego, not of the spirit. So, a simple step you can take is to close your eyes, focus on your love and gratitude for Tammy, and silently pray that to God. Say it to Tammy, too. 'Thank you. Thank you for your love and life.' Send her that love, fill your heart and home with it. If she's sensing you, I hope she'll know it's not a good idea to drop in until you're ready. When she does, it will likely be in a manner that has her signature written all over it. Something connected to who she was, and how she loved."

"Well, she did. She was a mom, loved her kids, so maybe that's why she tripped the toy in the nursery."

"You might be right. In that case, send the love, tell her you got the message, and then tell her, as only a sister can, to buzz off until you're ready!" We laughed, realizing that if God talks to us all the time, then why not our loved ones who've passed on? In the church we're encouraged to pray to the saints, to ask for intercession, to receive guidance. Why would that not more easily come through those who have personally loved and known us?

MOST OF THESE VISITS OCCUR AT THE DEATHBED, EITHER A FEW DAYS before or at the moment of death. For the patient, they are mostly very comforting. I recall one which was marked by the understandable confusion as reality shifted. Mike had been awaiting his death for months, and now with the advanced disease rendering him bed-bound and weak, it seemed the time was drawing close. Mike was one of those people I call "teachers," those patients who approach death with inspiring faith and love. He had an enviable equanimity, a profound peace, and a gracious and calm character. Though he could barely open his eyes, he was still one to joke with the staff. When asked how he was one morning, Mike gasped and faked death with a wry smile, and then couldn't help but chuckle as the nurse and family were caught by his dark humor.

I had the privilege of visiting the day after Mike had one of those experiences we all hear about but wonder if they're real. Not one but three of his deceased relatives came to visit. His mother told me the story, as Mike's mouth sores made it difficult to talk.

"It was like a wind breathing upon him. Then they were there: my husband and Mike's brother. They had all died years ago. It's so comforting to know they're all right. I can't tell you how much that means to me. Mike said they looked the best they did in this life!" (Even in heaven, relatives are reported to appear as they were in their prime.) "It was funny, though. Mike heard his brother say to his dad, 'He's sleeping. Let's not wake him.' His dad said, 'Of course he's sleeping, don't matter. He sees us.'" And Mike felt so calm, knowing who they were. Then, my sister, who was a nurse and died several years ago, comes in from the doorway. Mike looked at her and said, 'You're not my nurse!' She just turned around and left. Strange. But he felt real calm, it wasn't scary. Real comforting."

What was this visit for? Unlike an angelic or familiar visitation at death, they were not there to escort Mike to the other side but to give assurance so he won't be anxious when he does go. That, we knew, would be within a week or two. And we all wondered if we would be there to witness the next visit and get a glimpse of the other side waiting for us as well.

I sit quietly in my office after these conversations, wondering what those who've died are experiencing now and recalling the intensity and joy of my own glimpse of heaven. As I am exposed regularly to death and spiritual phenomena, I can't help but reflect on what I would have seen if I had reached the crest of that hill. What adventures await us? One thing is for sure: we'll all find out eventually!

IF WE'RE GOING REACH THAT OTHER SHORE, IF WE'RE GOING TO LOVE well, we're going to be broken. Perhaps grief is the signal that one's soul has made the evolutionary leap from potential to actualized immortality, for, as noted, grief is the price we pay for love. The wound of love is what Jesus willingly entered, what Karen beautifully practiced with Richard, what we are called to become. How we long for a miracle solution, when what's better is a miraculous incarnation. How we long to move beyond surviving, yet are terrified to do so.

Even in your grief, you are the very presence of God. You are weeping as Jesus wept. Yours is the body of Christ, yours are the hands extending heaven's love, yours are the lips speaking compassion and forgiveness, yours are the eyes witnessing the suffering of this world, and you can know the peace and presence as you offer your love as an instrument of God's love. It will be made complete in you. And it is the most powerful way you can participate in a wondrous enterprise: to be part of God's experience.

The idea that the experience of the universe adds to God's experience is difficult for many, let alone that each of us participates in this. It brings new meaning to the concept of a living God. It holds the paradox of being absolute and complete, yet also growing. This is the claim of process theology and quantum theology — modern expressions in the ancient struggle to articulate for each era the mystery of who God is and who we are becoming. These perspectives imply a partnership between God and sentient beings, between God and us. A foolish notion, given our track record. A beautiful notion, given the tapestry of life. A staggering notion that postulates God is evolving, expanding, growing through the experience of creation — perfection forever enriched, entangled, engaged.

Perhaps a better notion is that God is not so much evolving as expressing Godself. This creation, slowly yet relentlessly creeping toward Omega, is the means by which God manifests divine art — life itself. And the universe(s?) is entwined in a process by which the whole of creation will become self-aware, as God is. After all, spiritual evolution is a process that begins with the most elementary of particles and continues with beings like you and me — self-aware, able to love, to comprehend, to conceive that there is a God.

I wonder how it first happened. Imagine some primal hominid gazing out at the heavens, shining brighter than any starlit night we might be lucky enough to find. Moved by the grandeur of it all, this being realizes its insignificance, and yet, looking upon its family, feels an instinctive love that can stand in the face of an infinity of stars. This primate's awareness of the *mysterium tremendum* results in a new birth: the mortal being becomes a spiritual being. Love, which began as an evolutionary development, through which we build and maintain community, fidelity, and meaning, becomes something infinitely greater.

CHAPTER 19

GOING HOME

*Just like a sunbeam can't separate itself from the sun, and a wave can't
separate itself from the ocean, we can't separate ourselves from one another.
We are all part of a vast sea of love, one indivisible divine mind.*

— MARIANNE WILLIAMSON

AT DEATH THE BOND OF SINEW AND SOUL IS BROKEN. JUST AS WITH
any chemical reaction, something is released: energy — consciousness, the catalyst that facilitated a new structure through its presence in
the process, yet remained unchanged in its fundamental nature — being
eternal. Divine consciousness introduces flesh and spirit to each other
and seals the bond through love to birth a new entity, one self-aware,
itself able to become loving as its source — a child of God. But that will
take a while. Sometimes it takes eternity.

All spiritual traditions explore this. It is the hero's journey, the monomyth or singular story that captures the universal experience of growth
through suffering. To become the hero of your own life, you must leave
the comfort of hearth, home, and health, journey toward the danger (cancer, treatment), meeting mentors and allies along the way (your healthcare team, fellow patients). You have everything you need to do battle,
but it never feels like enough. You seek training (Google? A cancer coach?

A chaplain!) as you wrestle with the challenges, obstacles, and the ultimate fear — death. Done well, you engage with the suffering to realize unknown strength. Done poorly, you just postpone the homework. Most painful to discover: it is only through injury, and ultimately death, that the ultimate transformation comes.

An ancient myth that illustrates this paradox of suffering and hope is found in the Greek legend of Pandora's box. It is a psychological allegory of our journey toward authenticity, which parallels the Hebrew story of Eve and the transformative power of distressing NDEs. For the Greeks, Pandora was the first woman on Earth, created with water and soil. Among the gods under Zeus's reign were two brothers, Prometheus (meaning foresight) and Epimetheus (meaning hindsight). Prometheus stole fire from heaven, and brought it to earth. In vengeance (Greek gods were an emotional lot!), Zeus gave Pandora to Epimetheus in marriage and presented her with a beautiful gift, a container that she was never to open, for it contained all evil (or the shadow aspects of our psyche). Of course, you can predict what happened. Pandora opened it, and the contents escaped into the world, except for one thing that lay at the bottom of the jar: the Spirit of Hope.

It's a fascinating expression of the only way we are able to reach our most noble qualities — by first taking the lid off the darkness so that it is no longer contained, controlled, locked down.[165] Pandora becomes the instrument of a truly authentic humanity, although she, like Eve, is presented throughout history as the instrument of deception instead of awareness. It's another example of how, collectively, we push back against those who threaten our illusions of who we think we are.

In the face of death, our emotional wounds become either afflictions or affections: afflictions if they contain the dominant script by which we have played out our lives, affections as we are able to forgive, and use these painful passages to elevate our compassion for ourselves, for others, for the whole drama in which we have played a part. Pandora's curiosity was the key — she had to take a look. If we can also let curiosity lead us and compassion guide us, then we can take the lid off the things we have been suppressing and learn what they have been saying about our worthiness, our capacity to love and be loved, and how fear had led us away from that primary purpose. By so using cancer to become the hero of our own lives, we move beyond surviving to consciously evolving in love. There is no greater goal.

Imagine being able, along with St. Paul, to astonishingly describe even dying as a "momentary slight affliction." I am so privileged to witness those who embody that grace more than they can comprehend, souls who maintain an open heart, who radiate such a beautiful light. They never realize how they are teaching us, day by day, that gratitude is stronger than grief, praise is stronger than pain, and love is stronger than death. This is an ancient hope, recorded in 2 Corinthians, 4:14–18. When you are frail from fighting cancer and your body is a ghost of what was, these words are immense:

> [W]e know that the one who raised the Lord Jesus will raise us also with Jesus, and will bring us with you into his presence. Yes, everything is for your sake, so that grace, as it extends to more and more people, may increase thanksgiving, to the glory of God. So we do not lose heart. Even though our outer nature is wasting away, our inner nature is being renewed day by day. For this slight momentary affliction is preparing us for an eternal weight of glory beyond all measure, because we look not at what can be seen but at what cannot be seen; for what can be seen is temporary, but what cannot be seen is eternal.

It is this faith that sustains me in my work, walking into the greatest mystery, into the scariest times of people's lives, to bring the peace of God to them in gentle ways.

I never know what will happen, so I start each morning with a simple prayer: "Love through me." Then, with anticipation and assurance that I am supported by celestial beings and divine grace, I stumble into my day, fumble through my words, and am humbled as I encounter the hope that whispers to us all; the quantum whisper, such a delicate playing of the strings of life that it cannot be reduced to concrete assurance for the mind but resonates with the poetry of life in the heart. It reminds us that, as hard as life may be, we are never alone, and we never end.

When I hear of that resonance from families and patients, it piques my curiosity, my memory of what I glimpsed, and my anticipation of what is to come. While my soul literally dances with excitement whenever that thin veil is lifted, there's a whole new level of wonder when it happens in your own family, as it did recently with mine. This left the lot of us laughing and smiling in amazement, especially since it began so long ago, in 1975 near a place called Paradise, Nova Scotia.

BRIAN WAS THE YOUNGEST OF FIVE CHILDREN, LIVING IN THE IDYLLIC COMmunity of Grand Pré, an area blessed with rich soil and striking views of the Bay of Fundy's record tides. His parents, Norman, who was a professor of economics at Acadia University, and Sybil, gardened on the nine-acre property, raised German shepherds, and established one of the first vineyards that would evolve into a new industry in the area. It was a rich and wonderful life, but one marked, as most stories are, with a challenge that amplified their love even as it burdened their hearts. Brian was severely disabled.

From birth to death, he needed constant care. Parents and siblings fed him and dressed him, bathed him and transported him from bed to chair for all of his seventeen years. Although caring for Brian presented daily challenges, they loved him dearly, and gave him a life well beyond the doctor's prognosis.

Sybil filled the house with music, encouraging the family to gather at the piano for carols and tunes, or gently rendering Franz Liszt's *Liebesträume No.3* in the evening light; the title means "dreams of love," and was a favorite of hers. The last of the three romantic movements depicts unconditional love, perhaps expressing in melodic cadence what this mother's heart felt for her children, for her son who would occasionally sit under the piano, enveloped by vibration and sound. It was a way she could reach him beyond words, for his communication was severely limited. Still, they knew when he was happy, and they knew he belonged with them. He was dearly loved, and he loved in return from his own inner world. And then, all too soon, he left this one.

Brian died peacefully. His body was taken to the cemetery near Paradise, a place infused with stillness, presence, and beauty. It lies in a verdant valley with majestic elms, apple orchards, and rolling fields of wheat and corn. Buried with him was the weight of care. Left behind were the questions of life: Why do we suffer? What is the purpose? How can such hardship also be beautiful? These were quietly wrestled to the secret room of grief we all build, and life went on as normal. Until one day, when Norman had a visit from his son.

It was mid-day, a year after Brian's death. Norman was taking a break from his papers, sitting in his rocking chair next to the stereo. The recording was Dvořák's *New World Symphony*. He closed his eyes and leaned back as the opening chords of the second movement began, filled with hope and promise. Strings quietly introduced the familiar melody, then a solitary English horn carried the tune to his heart. The lyrics, added after Dvořák's time, moved through his mind:

> Goin' home. Goin' home. I'm a-goin' home.
> Quiet-like some still day, I'm just goin' home.
> It's not far, just close by, through an open door.
> Work all done, cares laid by, goin' to roam no more;
> Mother's there 'xpecting me, father's waiting, too,
> Lots of folks gathered there, all the friends I knew.

Something shifted. There was a slight crackling sound, he opened his eyes, and there before him was Brian. Brian, but not the son he knew. This young man was standing, he was strong, and oh, most glorious, he was smiling. Brian was more than well, he was whole and happy and very aware of his father's love. Norman began to rise, to speak, to extend his hand … then Brian was gone. Heart pounding, Norman's eyes searched through air still charged from the vision.

He told one of his daughters, Marg, months later. He told her of the day his heart was healed, the day he knew that all would be well. Perhaps, like most, Norman doubted it as the dream of love, all the while holding to the hope that it was, indeed, real. That would not be known for sure until thirty-one years later, when Norman, too, passed from this world. Once again the family gathered, once again the poetry of life whispered from the quantum realm. At the end of the service, as the family exited the sanctuary, the organist spontaneously began the familiar hymn, "Goin' home. Goin' home. I'm a-goin' home." Coincidence? It could have easily been brushed off as nothing more than a lucky alignment. After all, such a common hymn for a funeral. Still, it left Marg stunned. Could their father be telling them that he and Brian were together again?

Another seven years passed by, and Sybil's life had not turned out as she had hoped. The retirement home had been no replacement for those days of family under one roof and vitality in the bones. What remained were aches, both of the heart and the body, along with memories distorted by desire for what seemed like better days. She spent her time drawing flowers and birds, eating less, and sleeping more, until, with family at her side, she faded from this world.

The funeral celebrated Sybil through stories shared by her children, among them the memories of music in the home, in particular Liszt's *Liebesträume No. 3*. It seemed only fitting that afterwards we should gather at the old homestead, now a thriving winery, and raise a glass or two in her honor. We walked the property, sharing stories and looking out over the vineyard to the hill they used to toboggan down, and to the cliffs of Blomidon in the distance. The sun was low, and stomachs were growling, so we retired to the winery's restaurant to dine and reflect on the family's time together on the property so many years ago. And then, it happened again. Music. *Liebesträume*, third movement. Eyes went wide, mouths agape as we looked at each other in amazement. The room was quiet when we entered, there was no recording playing in the background, but then this gift floated through the air, not fifty feet from where the piano once stood. It felt as though Sybil was playing for her children once again, connecting with them through the ethereal power of music. We felt comforted knowing that she was with Norman and Brian in Paradise.

It would be enough for the story to end there. It seems, though, that Norman had one more thing to say. Several days after the funeral, Marg traveled out of the country to join her husband who was performing at a summer classical music festival. The first concert after her arrival was held in a large, open-air tent. It was a beautiful summer afternoon. After the brief intermission, she sat quietly, anxiously awaiting the featured work on the program. And then, of all the works in the vast orchestral repertoire that could have been chosen for this particular concert, the one piece began that resonated in Marg's soul with the signature of her father and brother: Dvořák's *New World Symphony*. The English horn brought tears to her eyes, and also a visitor unique among the 2000 audience members: a dragonfly. It lit upon a large yellow rose of her floral print dress. (A yellow rose was the logo for the nursing home that cared for Sybil in her final year, and these creatures had long been a symbol of resurrection and transformation for Marg.) There it remained, gazing into her eyes for almost a minute, slowly clapping its wings together in quiet applause. It seemed to portray a light-hearted joy, such a contrast to Marg's feelings of deep sadness. Thoughts of her mother intensified as she gazed back at the tiny creature perched on her knee. As the familiar melody floated to her ears, her parents' assurance enfolded her heart; they were together, all of them, and always will be.

> Morning star lights the way, restless dream all done.
> Shadows gone, break of day, real life just begun.
> There's no break, there's no end, just a living on;
> Wide awake, with a smile, going on and on.
> Going home. Going home, I'm just going home.
> It's not far, just close by, through an open door.

EPILOGUE

I ALWAYS WONDER WHAT THE JOURNEY WILL BRING FOR PATIENTS AF-
ter they leave our care. It is a profound comfort to meet them by chance
years later, to embrace and smile, exchanging a few words marked by deep
awareness of the gift of life.

I saw the wife of the Wiccan patient several years later. Her grief had
been profound, and her son had grown to be a fine young man, now in
medical school. Life had also brought her good things. Chief among them
was another chance at love. She had wondered if she would ever know a
love like she had and, as is often the case, the answer was no. She could
never repeat what was shared, but could grow into new love, new experiences, and new aspects of herself. What a wonderful surprise! And all the
love she had known was fuel for the journey.

Liz remained in our care and continued to be at peace with herself,
forgiving the past and incarnating a grace her father never could fully
understand. She used cancer for the healing of her heart, and died in
peace at the hospital in the quiet of the night. The nurse was by her side,
but no family.

I ran into Sam, two years after his transplant. He was even stronger
than before, had attained his seventh-level dan black belt, expanded his
martial arts school, and literally beamed with light and energy.

Bob also thrives and shines. His brilliant mind and artistry are enhanc-
ing lives around the world through the bionic braces he designs, which
increase strength and endurance for athletes and the injured alike. He continues to keep his body in peak form, and in my drawer is an eight-inch

nail he bent with his bare hands. (Makes me wonder if he is secretly working on other bionic enhancements.)

Doug continues to defy prognosis. Though the orb of energy, which gave him strength in the ICU, has never reappeared, he moves into his days confident that his journey is far from over. Doug finished his chemo and returned to work as a trucker. His divorce was finalized in his favor, finances improved, and life seems to have taken a turn for the better.

Steven, the young father who received the transplant from his brother, is doing well. The doctors decided to try the Dana Farber protocol, a two-year chemotherapy regime that was a shot in the dark. They had given him weeks to live, and when the spirits of his grandmothers and aunt had visited his father, John, with the message that they would give him strength, I thought they were saying Steven was going to die, that they would be with him and receive him. I've never been so happy to be wrong. Steven's son is growing like a weed, and though they continue to work on the Camaros in the garage, the cars are still not running properly.

It was difficult asking Josh's parents' permission to share his story. The loss of a child is sacred ground in the heart, and I fretted for days before sending the request. When we did connect, it was infused with divine synchronicity and guidance. His father shared that the day Josh died, he went to the chapel to pray that Josh would be at peace, that he would not be afraid as he died, that he would feel their love. Thirteen years later, my request arrived with the story, describing my sense that Josh felt exactly that. Thirteen years later, he knew his prayer had been answered.

His mother had not discussed their loss in years, but just that week was chatting with friends about the concept of an energetic anatomy. She shared with them the difference Therapeutic Touch made to her son. Then my request arrived. She had no doubt her son was guiding our encounter, and watches over them.

And me? My health continues to be good, and I continue in my journey, an exploration of the nature of consciousness and the staggering wisdom of God's love.

END NOTES

PREFACE

1. Suzanne H. Reuben, *Reducing Environmental Cancer Risk: What We Can Do Now* (Darby, PA: DIANE Publishing, 2010).

CHAPTER 1

2. "Paraganglioma," Wikipedia, accessed January 2, 2016, https://en.wikipedia.org/wiki/Paraganglioma. Original source unknown.
3. https://www.uclahealth.org/endocrine-center/pheochromocytoma-treatment-and-diagnosis accessed January 2, 2016.

CHAPTER 2

4. "Common Cancer Types," National Cancer Institute, updated February 1, 2016, www.cancer.gov/types/common-cancers.
5. Canadian Cancer Society and Government of Canada, *Canadian Cancer Statistics 2015*, May 2015, adapted June 2015, 16, www.cancer.ca/~/media/cancer.ca/CW/cancer%20information/cancer%20101/Canadian%20cancer%20statistics/Canadian-Cancer-Statistics-2015-EN.pdf.
6. Wael Saber, Shaun Opie, J. Douglas Rizzo, Mei-Jie Zhang, Mary M. Horowitz, and Jeff Schriber. "Outcomes After Matched Unrelated Donor Versus Identical Sibling Hematopoietic Cell Transplantation in Adults with Acute Myelogenous Leukemia." *Blood* 119, no. 17 (2012): 3908–16.
7. Jinchuan Hu, Sheera Adar, Christopher P. Selby, Jason D. Lieb, and Aziz Sancar, "Genome-Wide Analysis of Human Global and Transcription-Coupled Excision Repair of UV Damage at Single-Nucleotide Resolution," *Genes & Development* 29, no. 9 (2015): 948–60.
8. Robert M. Hoffman, "Application of GFP Imaging in Cancer," *Laboratory Investigation* 95, no. 4 (2015): 432–52.
9. Mee Rie Sheen, Patrick H. Lizotte, Seiko Toraya-Brown, and Steven Fiering, "Stimulating Antitumor Immunity with Nanoparticles," *Wiley Interdisciplinary Reviews: Nanomedicine and Nanobiotechnology* 6, no. 5 (2014): 496–505.
10. Enming Zhang, Moritz F. Kircher, Martin Koch, Lena Eliasson, S. Nahum Goldberg, and Erik Renström, "Dynamic Magnetic Fields Remote-Control Apoptosis via Nanoparticle Rotation," *ACS Nano* 8, no. 4 (2014): 3192–201.

11. Freddie Bray, Ahmedin Jemal, Nathan Grey, Jacques Ferlay, and David Forman, "Global Cancer Transitions According to the Human Development Index (2008–2030): A Population-Based Study," *The Lancet Oncology* 13, no. 8 (2012): 790–801.

CHAPTER 3
12. Karen Armstrong, *A History of God* (New York: Ballantine, 1994), 383.

CHAPTER 4
13. Joann Hungelmann, Eileen Kenkel-Rossi, Loretta Klassen, and Ruth Stollenwerk. "Focus on Spiritual Well-Being: Harmonious Interconnectedness of Mind-Body-Spirit – Use of the JAREL Spiritual Well-Being Scale: Assessment of Spiritual Well-Being is Essential to the Health of Individuals," *Geriatric Nursing* 17, no. 6 (1996): 262–66.
14. Centers for Disease Control and Prevention, "Autism Spectrum Disorder," last update July 2016, http://www.cdc.gov/ncbddd/autism/data.html.
15. Colin D. Mathers, and Dejan Loncar, "Projections of Global Mortality and Burden of Disease from 2002 to 2030," *Plos med* 3, no. 11 (2006): e442.
16. Ahmedin Jemal, Melissa M. Center, Carol DeSantis, and Elizabeth M. Ward, "Global Patterns of Cancer Incidence and Mortality Rates and Trends," *Cancer Epidemiology Biomarkers & Prevention* 19, no. 8 (2010): 1893–1907.
17. L. D. Leffall and M. L. Kripke, "President's Cancer Panel: Reducing Environmental Cancer Risk," *National Cancer Institute* (2010).
18. Ahmedin Jemal, 1893–1907.
19. Preetha Anand, Ajaikumar B. Kunnumakara, Chitra Sundaram, Kuzhuvelil B. Harikumar, Sheeja T. Tharakan, Oiki S. Lai, Bokyung Sung, and Bharat B. Aggarwal, "Cancer Is a Preventable Disease that Requires Major Lifestyle Changes," *Pharmaceutical Research* 25, no. 9 (2008): 2097–116.
20. World Cancer Research Fund / American Institute for Cancer Research, *Food, Nutrition, Physical Activity, and the Prevention of Cancer: a Global Perspective*, Washington DC: AICR, 2007.
21. Jonathan M. Samet, Erika Avila-Tang, Paolo Boffetta, Lindsay M. Hannan, Susan Olivo-Marston, Michael J. Thun, and Charles M. Rudin, "Lung Cancer in Never Smokers: Clinical Epidemiology and Environmental Risk Factors," *Clinical Cancer Research* 15, no. 18 (2009): 5626–645.
22. Vini G. Khurana, Charles Teo, Michael Kundi, Lennart Hardell, and Michael Carlberg, "Cell Phones and Brain Tumors: A Review Including the Long-Term Epidemiologic Data," *Surgical Neurology* 72, no. 3 (2009): 205–14.

23. Oakley Ray, "How the Mind Hurts and Heals the Body," *American Psychologist* 59, no. 1 (2004): 29.

24. Franco Merletti, Claudia Galassi, and Teresa Spadea. "The Socioeconomic Determinants of Cancer." *Environ Health* 10, no. Suppl 1 (2011): S7.

25. Ray Kurzweil, The Singularity Is Near: When Humans Transcend Biology Penguin, New York, (2005). For weekly updates visit http://www.kurzweilai.net

26. Kenneth I. Pargament, Bruce W. Smith, Harold G. Koenig, and Lisa Perez, "Patterns of Positive and Negative Religious Coping with Major Life Stressors," *Journal for the Scientific Study of Religion* 37 (1998): 710–24.

CHAPTER 5

27. Gabriel S. Dy-Liacco, Ralph L. Piedmont, Nichole A. Murray-Swank, Thomas E. Rodgerson, and Martin F. Sherman, "Spirituality and Religiosity as Cross-cultural Aspects of Human Experience," *Psychology of Religion and Spirituality* 1, no. 1 (2009): 35.

28. Kenneth I. Pargament and Patrick J. Sweeney, "Building Spiritual Fitness in the Army: An Innovative Approach to a Vital Aspect of Human Development," *American Psychologist* 66, no. 1 (2011): 58.

29. Cassandra Vieten, Shelley Scammell, Ron Pilato, Ingrid Ammondson, Kenneth I. Pargament, and David Lukoff, "Spiritual and Religious Competencies for Psychologists." *Psychology of Religion and Spirituality* 5, no. 3 (2013): 129.

30. Rudolf Otto, *The Idea of the Holy* 14 (New York: Oxford University Press, 1958).

31. Rob Bell, *NOOMA Breathe | 014*, (Flannel: 2006), 14:47.

CHAPTER 6

32. Alexander Shifrin, "Pheochomocytoma," The Adrenal Gland Tumours, 2012, accessed February 22, 2015, www.adrenaltumors.org/Pheochromocytoma.

33. American Association for Physicians and Surgeons, Inc., "Physician Oaths," accessed February 22, 2015, http://www.aapsonline.org/ethics/oaths.htm.

CHAPTER 7

34. Andrea Parrot and Nina Cummings, *Forsaken Females: The Global Brutalization of Women* (Lanham, MD: Rowman & Littlefield, 2006).

35. Ellen Bass and Laura David, *The Courage to Heal: A Guide for Women Survivors of Sexual Abuse*, 3rd ed. (New York: Harper and Row, 1988), 24.

36. An excellent commentary and reading, along with the entire poem, can be found at Maria Popova, "Love After Love: Derek Walcott's Poetic Ode to Being at Home in Ourselves," brainpickings, accessed September 30, 2016, http://www.brainpickings.org/2015/04/21/love-after-love-derek-walcott/.

37. Parker J. Palmer, *A Hidden Wholeness: The Journey toward an Undivided Life.* (Hoboken, NJ: John Wiley & Sons, 2009).

CHAPTER 8

38. Kahlil Gibran, *The Prophet* (Ware, Hertfortshire: Wordsworth Editions, 1996), 16.

39. George A. Bonanno, *The Other Side of Sadness: What the New Science of Bereavement Tells Us About Life after Loss* (New York: Basic Books, 2009).

40. Derek Thompson, "The Secret Life of Grief: My Mom's Cancer and the Science of Resilience, *The Atlantic*, December 3, 2013, www.theatlantic.com/health/archive/2013/12/the-secret-life-of-grief/281992/.

41. Ibid.

42. William Shakespeare, *Hamlet*, Act 3, scene 1, *The Riverside Shakespeare*, ed. G. Blakemore Evans (Boston: Houghton Mifflin, 1974) 1160.

43. Lee Ellis, Eshah A. Wahab, and Malini Ratnasingan, "Religiosity and Fear of Death: A Three Nation Comparison," *Mental Health, Religion & Culture* 16, no. 2 (2013): 179–99.

44. A powerful guide in dying not only well but also beautifully is *Being With Dying: Cultivating Compassion and Fearlessness in the Presence of Death* by Joan Halifax: (Shambhala Publications, 2008).

45. Matthew O'Reilly, "'Am I dying?' The Honest Answer," TED.com, filmed July 2014, accessed April 12, 2014, www.ted.com/talks/matthew_o_reilly_am_i_dying_the_honest_answer.

CHAPTER 9

46. Brené Brown, "The Power of Vulnerability," filmed June 2010, accessed October 3, 2016, https://www.ted.com/talks/brene_brown_on_vulnerability?language=en.

47. Ibid.

48. Linda Carlson, Tom Baker, and Joan Halifax, "Chapter 8: Mindfulness for Cancer and Terminal Illness," Harvard University, accessed October 14, 2014, http://isites.harvard.edu/fs/docs/icb.topic1451261.files/Core%20Readings.pdf.

49. Lesley Hazleton, "On Reading the Koran," TED.com, filmed October 2010, accessed October 12, 2016, www.ted.com/talks/lesley_hazelton_on_reading_the_koran?language=en.

50. Pema Chödrön, *The Shenpa Syndrome*, 2006, accessed January 1, 2016, http://deoxy.org/wiki/action=browse&id=Shenpa&raw=2

CHAPTER 10

51. Dr. Ian Gawler, "Remarkable Recoveries: Surviving Cancer Against the Odds. What are the chances? How is it done?" (public address, May 2008), http://iangawler.com/info/articles/Remarkable%20Recoveries.pdf; also, see "Frequently Asked Questions about Spontaneous Remissions," Institute of Noetic Sciences, http://www.noetic.org/research/project/spontaneous-remission/faqs.

52. Caryle Hirshberg and Marc Barasch, *Remarkable Recovery: What Extraordinary Healings Tell Us About Getting Well and Staying Well* (New York: Riverhead Books, 1995).

53. Cara Feinberg. "The Placebo Phenomenon," *Harvard Magazine* (2013): 36–39.

54. "Injury Prevention and Control: Division of Violence Protection," Centers for Disease Control and Prevention, last updated January 2014, http://www.cdc.gov/violenceprevention/pub/healthy_infants.html.

55. Alastair J. Cunningham and Kimberly Watson, "How Psychological Therapy May Prolong Survival in Cancer Patients: New Evidence and a Simple Theory," *Integrative Cancer Therapies* 3, no. 3 (2004): 214–29.

56. Marcus Alexander and Nicholas A. Christakis, "Bias and Asymmetric Loss in Expert Forecasts: A Study of Physician Prognostic Behavior with Respect to Patient Survival," *Journal of Health Economics* 27, no. 4 (2008): 1095–108.

57. Mark 5:30–34.

58. For a wonderful exploration of this, watch Rob Bell's video "Rhythm," released 2005, https://flannel.org/products/nooma-rhythm-011.

CHAPTER 11

59. Peter Sedlmeier et al., "The Psychological Effects of Meditation: A Meta-Analysis," *Psychological Bulletin* 138, no. 6 (2012): 113.

60. Robert H. Schneider et al., "Stress Reduction in the Secondary Prevention of Cardiovascular Disease Randomized, Controlled Trial of Transcendental Meditation and Health Education in Blacks," *Circulation: Cardiovascular Quality and Outcomes* 5, no. 6 (2012): 750–58.

61. Ursula K. Le Guin, *The Wave in the Mind: Talks and Essays on the Writer, the Reader, and the Imagination.* (Boston: Shambhala Publications, 2004).

Chapter 12

62. John 14:13. Unfortunately, this instruction has been reduced to a formula in the church. We now tag His name onto the end of a prayer, "This we ask for in the name of Jesus Christ, our Lord," as if that gives a stamp of delivery. However, to ask in the name of someone means to ask in the same character of that person, in the spirit of everything that name represents. In other words, to be one with the consciousness of Christ.

63. Edward F. Kelly, Emily Williams Kelly, Adam Crabtree, Alan Gauld, Michael Grosso, and Bruce Greyson, *Irreducible Mind: Toward a Psychology for the 21st Century* (Lanham, MD: Rowman & Littlefield, 2007).

64. Ankur Jhaveri et al., "Therapeutic Touch Affects DNA Synthesis and Mineralization of Human Osteoblasts in Culture," *Journal of Orthopaedic Research* 26, no. 11 (November 2008): 1541–546.

65. Marie Giasson and Louise Bouchard, "Effect of Therapeutic Touch on the Well-Being of Persons with Terminal Cancer," *Journal of Holistic Nursing* 16, no. 3 (September 1998): 383–98.

66. Dolores Krieger, *The Therapeutic Touch: How to Use Your Hands to Help or to Heal*, 1st ed. (New York: Prentice Hall Press, 1986).

67. Dolores Krieger, *Accepting Your Power to Heal: The Personal Practice of Therapeutic Touch* (Rochester, VT: Inner Traditions/Bear & Co, 1993), 7.

68. National Cancer Institute, "Managing Chemotherapy Side Effects: Nausea and Vomiting," revised February 2012, http://www.cancer.gov/publications/patient-education/nausea.pdf, 1.

69. Hui-Fu Guo et al., "Brain Substrates Activated by Electroacupuncture of Different Frequencies (I): Comparative Study on the Expression of Oncogene C-Fos and Genes Coding for Three Opioid Peptides," *Molecular Brain Research* 43, no. 1 (January 1997): 157–66.

70. MultiWaveResearch, "Multi Wave Research," 2010–2015, accessed November 24, 2015, http://users.skynet.be/Lakhovsky/Getting%20Started.htm.

71. Vlail P. Kaznacheyev, S. P. Shurin, L. P. Mikhailova, and N. V. Ignatovish, "Distant Intercellular Interactions in a System of Two Tissue Cultures," *Psychoenergetic Systems* 1, no. 3 (1976): 141–42.

72. Raymond S. Burr, *Blueprint for Immortality: The Electrical Patterns of Life* (London, UK: Neville Spearman, 1972), 95

73. Victor Guillemin, *The Story of Quantum Mechanics* (Mineola, NY: Courier Corporation, 1968).

74. H. S. Burr and F. S. C. Northrop, "The Electro-Dynamic Theory of Life," *Quarterly Review of Biology* 10, no. 3 (September 1935):322–33.

75. We will explore shortly how the universe arises from consciousness, that it, astonishingly, exists only in your mind.

76. S. J. Swithenby, "SQUID Magnetometers: Uses in Medicine," *Physics in Technology* 18, no. 1 (1987): 17.

77. William T. Joines, Stephen B. Baumann, and John G. Kruth, "Electromagnetic Emission from Humans During Focused Intent," *The Journal of Parapsychology* 76, no. 2 (2012): 275.

78. Robert O. Becker, Charles H. Bachman, and Howard Friedman, "The Direct Current Control System. A Link Between Environment and Organism," *New York State Journal of Medicine* 62 (April 15, 1962): 1169–176.

79. David L. Nelson, Bob M. Cox, and Albert L. Lehninger, *Principles of Biochemistry*, 5th ed. (New York: Worth Publishers, 2000), 744.

80. Amy S. Chuong et al., "Noninvasive Optical Inhibition with a Red-Shifted Microbial Rhodopsin," *Nature Neuroscience* 17, no. 8 (2014): 1123–129.

81. R. McCraty, M. Atkinson, and D. Tomasino, *Science of the Heart: Exploring the Role of the Heart in Human Performance* (Boulder Creek, CA: Institute of HeartMath, 2001).

82. Margaret Moga, "Magnetic Field Activity During Healing Sessions with Dr. Bengston," Healing with Intent (blog), February 10, 2015, www.indiana. edu/~brain/magnetic-field-activity-during-healing-sessions-with-dr-bengston/.

CHAPTER 13

83. Donald Franklin Moyer, "Revolution in Science: The 1919 Eclipse Test of General Relativity," in *On the Path of Albert Einstein*, ed. Arnold Perlmutter and Linda F. Scott (New York: Springer US, 1979), 55.

84. A method that is not as without bias or inconsistency as one might think. See Rupert Sheldrake, *The Science Delusion* (London, UK: Coronet, 2012). See also Rupert Sheldrake, "The Science Delusion," TEDxWhitechapel video, filmed January 12, 2013 accessed September 12, 2016, http://www. sheldrake.org/reactions/tedx-whitechapel-the-banned-talk.

85. Some philosophers and physicists will undoubtedly find it difficult to indulge my bias towards a spiritual explanation of consciousness. However, it is unapologetically presented with the caveat that just as there appears to be two sets of rules that govern the universe, classical and quantum physics, I believe there are two levels of reality, spiritual and physical. The physical level is a projection of consciousness; the Universe is the externalization of the soul. We who inhabit the finite (for now) will never be able to use our set of rules and perception to explain the infinite. However, the infinite can reveal itself to the finite, and does so by sustaining it in every moment.

86. Letter to Mersenne, November 25, 1630, found in Stephen Gaukroger, *Descartes: An Intellectual Biography* (New York: Oxford University Press, 1995).

87. Explore this through the work of Stuart Hammeroff and Roger Penrose, Quantum Consciousness, accessed October 3, 2016, at http://www.quantumconsciousness.org/.

88. W. W. Rouse Ball, *A Short Account of the History of Mathematic* (New York: Dover Publications, 1960).

89. Chaos theory is an excellent example, an astonishing demonstration of the interconnectedness of all things. It turns out the universe is governed by a beautiful set of mathematical principles that for some are deeply mystical in nature, without requiring a God to drive them. Of course, others see chaos theory as evidence of divine wisdom. Highly recommended is *The Secret Life of Chaos*, accessed October 4, 2016, http://www.dailymotion.com/video/xv1j0n_the-secret-life-of-chaos_shortfilms.

90. This does not mean the bigger the brain, the more advanced the consciousness. There is actually an optimal brain size for high-level consciousness, after which the time for neuronal transmission begins to slow due to sheer mass. We are in the optimal range, a whale is not.

CHAPTER 14

91. See Carl Sagan explain the story, accessed April 20, 2014, https://www.youtube.com/watch?v=rAAeLNAfSYc&nohtml5=False.

92. Edward F. Kelly et al., *Irreducible Mind.*

93. Dean Radin, *The Conscious Universe* (New York: HarperCollins Publishers, 1997). See also IONS Communications Team, "Psychic Abilities and the Illusion of Separation, accessed February 12, 2013, http://noetic.org/blog/communications-team/psychic-abilities-and.

94. The Global Consciousness Project, accessed February 12, 2013, see http://noosphere.princeton.edu/. For this experiment, researchers at Princeton University were granted the first US patent for a psi effect on November 3, 1998. Patent "US 5830064" is titled: "Apparatus and method for distinguishing events which collectively exceed chance expectations and thereby controlling an output. This patent specifically covers distant mental control of electronic random number generator outputs."

95. Roger Nelson, "The Global Consciousness Project: Formal Analysis September 11, 2001," 1998–2015, accessed February 12, 2013, http://global-mind.org/911formal.html.

96. Charles T. Tart, *The End of Materialism: How Evidence of the Paranormal is Bringing Science and Spirit Together* (Oakland, CA: Noetic Books, Institute of Noetic Sciences, New Harbinger Publications, 2009).

97. Uwe Wolfradt, "Dissociative Experiences, Trait Anxiety and Paranormal Beliefs," *Personality and Individual Differences* 23, no. 1 (July 1997): 15–19.

CHAPTER 16

98. Pim van Lommel, Ruud van Wees, Vincent Meyers, and Ingrid Elfferich, "Near-Death Experience in Survivors of Cardiac Arrest: A Prospective Study in the Netherlands," *The Lancet* 358, no. 9298 (2001): 2039–045.

99. James H. Lindley, Sethyn Bryan, and Bob Conley, "Near-Death Experiences in a Pacific Northwest American Population: The Evergreen Study," *Journal of Near Death Experiences* 1 (1981): 104–25.

100. Janice Minor Holden, Bruce Greyson, and Debbie James, eds., *The Handbook of Near-Death Experiences: Thirty Years of Investigation* (Santa Barbara, CA: Praeger/ABC-CLIO, 2009).

101. IANDS, "Key Facts About Near-Death Experiences," accessed October 16, 2016, http://iands.org/ndes/about-ndes/key-nde-facts21.html?start=2.

102. Kevin Williams, "Music and the Near-Death Experience," Near-Death Experiences and the Afterlife, accessed March 20, 2015, www.near-death.com/experiences/research29.html.

103. Brené Brown, *Listening to Shame,* TED Talk, filmed March 2012, accessed October 16, 2016, https://www.ted.com/talks/brene_brown_listening_to_shame?language=en

104. Explore more through the thousands of NDE cases dating from 1877 to the present day. See IANDS, "Index to NDE Periodical Literature," last updated May 20, 2015, http://iands.org/research/nde-research/index-to-nde-periodical-literature.html

105. Raymond A. Moody, *Glimpses of Eternity: An Investigation into Shared Death Experiences* (Nashville, TN: Random House, 2011).

106. Michael Barbato et al., "Parapsychological Phenomena Near the Time of Death," *Journal of Palliative Care* 15, no. 2 (1998): 30–37. See also Janice Holden et al., "Spontaneous Mediumship Experiences: A Neglected Aftereffect of Near-Death Experiences," *Journal of Near-Death Studies* 33, no. 2 (2014): 67-85.

107. May Eulitt, and Stephen Hoyer, *Fireweaver: The Story of a Life, a Near-Death, and Beyond* (Bloomington, IN: Xlibris Corporation, 2001).

108. Gregory Shushan, ed. *Conceptions of the Afterlife in Early Civilizations: Universalism, Constructivism and Near-Death Experience*, vol. 6 (London: UK: A&C Black, 2009).

109. Nancy Evans Bush, *Dancing Past the Dark: Distressing Near-Death Experiences* (BookBaby, 2012).

110. See Mark 12:28–31, Luke 10:25–37, John 13:34–35.

111. Bruce Greyson, "Near-Death Experiences Precipitated by Suicide Attempt: Lack of Influence of Psychopathology, Religion, and Expectations," *Journal of Near-Death Studies* 9, no. 3 (1991): 183–88. See also Ring, Kenneth, and Stephen Franklin. "Do suicide survivors report near-death experiences?." *OMEGA-Journal of Death and Dying* 12.3 (1982): 191-208, accessed January 2, 2017, http://journals.sagepub.com/doi/pdf/10.2190/47XB-EGMR-9WKP-H3BX

112. Kenneth Ring, *Life at Death: A Scientific Investigation of the Near-Death Experience* (New York: Coward McCann, 1980).

113. Bruce Greyson, and Nancy Evans Bush, "Distressing Near-Death Experiences," *Psychiatry* 55, no. 1 (1992): 95–110.

114. Nancy Evans Bush, "Untangling Hellish Visions," published December 9, 2012, accessed February 12, 2015, www.youtube.com/watch?v=8Gghhqcu-Es.

115. A. R. Turner, *The History of Hell* (New York: Harcourt Brace and Company, 1993), 102.

116. C. Zaleski, *Otherworld Journeys: Accounts of Near-Death Experience in Medieval and Modern Times* (New York: Oxford University Press, 1987), 149.

117. Joseph Campbell, *The Hero with a Thousand Faces* vol. 17 (Novato, CA: New World Library, 2008).

118. Not as overtly as I'm stating, of course. This is a theological reflection upon the experience — my musings, not NDE research.

119. Distressing NDEs closely match descriptions in *The Tibetan Book of the Dead*. See Samuel Bercholz, *A Guided Tour of Hell: A Graphic Memoir* (Boston: Shambhala Publications 2016).

120. Arjun Walia, "'Consciousness Creates Reality' — Physicists Admit the Universe Is Immaterial, Mental and Spiritual," posted November 11, 2014, accessed September 28, 2016, http://www.collective-evolution.com/2014/11/11/consciousness-creates-reality-physicists-admit-the-universe-is-immaterial-mental-spiritual/.

121. Arjun Bagchi, Rudranil Basu, Daniel Grumiller, and Max Riegler, "Entanglement Entropy in Galilean Conformal Field Theories and Flat Holography," *Physical Review Letters* 114, no. 11 (2015): 111602.

122. Maddie Stone, "There Is Growing Evidence that Our Universe Is a Giant Hologram"

123Published May 5, 2015, accessed September 28, 2016, http://motherboard. vice.com/en_ca/read/there-is-growing-evidence-that-our-universe-is-a-giant-hologram.

124. Lanza, Robert. "A new theory of the universe." *American Scholar* 76, no. 2 (2007): 18, accesses January 2, 2017, https://theamericanscholar.org/a-new-theory-of-the-universe/#

125. This is beautifully presented in the C. S. Lewis classic *The Great Divorce*. In this theological fantasy, he defines two types of people, those who say to God, "Thy will be done," and those to whom God says, in the end, "Thy will be done." The gates of hell are locked from the inside. Lewis, *The Great Divorce*, ed. Clive Staples (New York: Macmillan, 1946).

126. In Luke 16:19–31, Jesus speaks of a chasm dividing paradise and Sheol that is impossible to cross. That rescue has been experienced during distressing NDEs may indicate these experiences are more akin to the hero's journey experienced by mystics, than to the permanent state of death and whatever lies beyond. NDEs are, by definition, initial stages of a raw existential state, not permanent transformations into them.

127. C. Bache, "Expanding Grof's Concept of the Perinatal: Deepening the Inquiry into Frightening Near-Death Experiences," *Journal of Near-Death Studies* 15 (1996):113–39.

128. Our entire model of reality could actually be backwards. Instead of originating with the Big Bang and moving "forward" through time, the universe may "start" in this moment, with time built backwards from it. Explore this further with Robert Lanza, *Beyond Biocentrism: Rethinking Time, Space, Consciousness, and the Illusion of Death* (Dallas, TX: BenBella Books, 2016).

CHAPTER 17

129. Sam Parnia, D. G. Waller, Robert Yeates, and Peter Fenwick, "A Qualitative and Quantitative Study of the Incidence, Features and Aetiology of Near Death Experiences in Cardiac Arrest Survivors," *Resuscitation* 48, no. 2 (2001): 149–56.

130. Kenneth Ring, "Religious Wars in the NDE Movement: Some Personal Reflections on Michael Sabom's Light & Death.," *Journal of Near-Death Studies* 18, no. 4 (2000): 215–44.

131. Discovery Channel interview uploaded on October 26, 2009, at www. youtube.com/watch?v=Bu1ErDeQ0Zw.

132. Janice Miner Holden, Bruce Greyson, and Debbie James, eds., *The Handbook of Near-Death Experiences: Thirty Years of Investigation* (Santa Barbara, CA: Praeger/ABC-CLIO, 2009).

133. Olaf Blanke and Shahar Arzy, "The Out-of-Body Experience: Disturbed Self-Processing at the Temporo-Parietal Junction," *The Neuroscientist* 11, no. 1 (2005): 16–24.

134. Jimo Borjigin et al., "Surge of Neurophysiological Coherence and Connectivity in the Dying Brain," *Proceedings of the National Academy of Sciences* 110, no. 35 (2013): 14432–437.

135. Rebecca Morelle, "Near-Death Experiences and 'Electrical Surge in Dying Brain," BBC News, August 13, 2013, www.bbc.com/news/science-environment-23672150.

136. Bruce Greyson, "Differentiating Spiritual and Psychotic Experiences: Sometimes a Cigar Is Just a Cigar," *Journal of Near-Death Studies* 32 (2014): 123–36.

137. Peter Fenwick, "Science and Spirituality: A Challenge for the 21st Century," *Journal of Near-Death Studies* 23 (2004): 131–57.

138. Kat McGowan, "How Much of Your Memory is True?" Discover, August 3, 2009, accessed September 16, 2016, http://discovermagazine.com/2009/jul-aug/03-how-much-of-your-memory-is-true.

139. Natasha A. Tassell-Matamua, and Nicole Lindsay, "'I'm not Afraid to Die': the Loss of the Fear of Death After a Near-Death Experience," *Mortality* 21, no. 1 (2016): 71–87.

140. Bruce Greyson, "Near-Death Experiences and Spirituality," *Zygon* 41, no. 2 (2006): 393.

141. McGowan, "How Much of Your Memory is True?." .

142. Daniel Kahneman, "The Riddle of Experience vs. Memory," TED.com, filmed February 2010, accessed January 5, 2015, www.ted.com/talks/daniel_kahneman_the_riddle_of_experience_vs_memory/transcript?language=en#t-28729.

143. Marie Thonnard et al., "Characteristics of Near-Death Experiences Memories as Compared to Real and Imagined Events Memories," *PLOS one* 8, no. 3 (March 2013), accessed October 12, 2015, www.plosone.org/article/info:doi/10.1371/journal.pone.0057620.

144. Pam Kircher, "NDEs in the Medical Profession," International Association for Near Death Studies newsletter *Vital Signs* 20, no. 2 (2001), accessed December 14, 2014, http://iands.org/support/considerations-for-caregivers/ndes-and-medicine.html.

145. C. O. Monument, "Electromagnetic Phenomena Reported by Near-Death Experiencers," *Journal of Near-Death Studies* 33 (2015): 4.

146. More research is needed to verify this. Adult reports vary between 10and 40 percent, while in children it may be 70-plus percent. IANDS, "Children's

Near-Death Experiences," accessed October 6, 2016, http://iands.org/ndes/about-ndes/distressing-ndes.html#a3.

147. P. M. H. Atwater, *The New Children and Near-Death Experiences* (Rochester, VT: Inner Traditions/Bear & Co, 2003), 81–103.

148. Linda J. Griffith, "Near-Death Experiences and Psychotherapy," *Psychiatry MMC* 6, no. 10 (2009).

149. P. M. H. Atwater, "Aftereffects of Near-Death States," International Association for Near Death Studies, 1998, accessed December 14, 2013, http://iands.org/about-ndes/common-aftereffects.html.

150. Sandra Rozan Christian, "Marital Satisfaction and Stability Following a Near-Death Experience of One of the Marital Partners," (PhD diss., University of North Texas, 2005).

151. Bruce Greyson, "Near-Death Experience: Clinical Implications," *Archives of Clinical Psychiatry (São Paulo)* 34 (2007): 116–25.

152. Cherie Sutherland, "Changes in Religious Beliefs, Attitudes, and Practices Following Near-Death Experiences: An Australian Study," *Journal of Near-Death Studies* 9, no. 1 (1990): 21–31.

153. This is, in fact, the fourth letter he had written to Corinth. The account is first mentioned in 1 Corinthians 5:9, the second is the actual letter we call 1 Corinthians, and the third is mentioned in what we call 2 Corinthians, the fourth letter. (St. Paul is known for being somewhat complicated in his writing!)

154. Acts 22: 6-1. Saul's name changed to Paul, a common practice in ancient times to reflect a new spiritual identity and purpose in life.

155. 2 Corinthians 12:2–7.

156. 1 Corinthians 15:8–9.

157. 1 Corinthians 15: 40–49.

158. Philippians 1:21–24.

159. 1 Corinthians 13:1–12

160. Nina S. Kadan Lottick et al., "Psychiatric Disorders and Mental Health Service Use in Patients with Advanced Cancer," *Cancer* 104, no. 12 (2005): 2872–881.

161. Though there are cases of those who do attempt. They have such trouble adapting to this life again that they become dissatisfied with this world. Their lives are marked by a deep dissonance and homesickness for that ethereal state.

CHAPTER 18

162. Thomas Szasz, *The Second Sin* (New York: Doubleday, 1973), 101.

163. This is very much along the lines of *theosis* in the Eastern Orthodox Christian tradition. Through union of our consciousness with Christ, we take on, or resonate with, His divine likeness. We become God in divine energies or operations, but not in God's essence or identity.

164. Derek Flood, *Healing the Gospel: A Radical Vision for Grace, Justice, and the Cross* (Eugene, OR: Wipf and Stock Publishers, 2012). This excellent book explores the violent and oppressive conceptions of the crucifixion. Explore a summary at http://therebelgod.com/CrossPaper.pdf, accessed October 16, 2016.

CHAPTER 19

165. This also applies to NDEs, especially distressing ones. In that raw state of consciousness, the darkness is best received without repression or projection. Compassion integrates the estranged aspects of the self, leading to authenticity. The point, again, is not to be good, but to be real.

Acknowledgments

THIS BOOK HAD TO BE WRITTEN, THOUGH I RESISTED IT FOR OVER TEN years. It started sporadically, a story here and there, but gained momentum with a particularly heavy case: Josh from chapter 3. I woke at 4:00 a.m. and began, which would become my habit for two years. This was as much a form of therapy as it was a creative endeavor. Spiritual care is a profoundly meaningful vocation, and I am honored to provide support to so many, but suffering is meant to be fuel for transformation, and I had a lot to work with. To my patients, you likely never suspected that you were such teachers, helping me grow in faith and wonder through the years. To those of you who consented to have your stories included, I am especially grateful, and hope others are blessed by your courage and noble spirits.

Thank you to my good friend Freeman Patterson. Freeman, your feedback and encouragement were instrumental in setting my commitment to take this project seriously. Thank you for connecting me with Nina Denham. The two of you became my guides, reviewing each chapter and sifting my thoughts. It seemed you were heaven-sent, literally. I could not have done this without you.

Thank you to my editor, Paula Sarson. Paula, I handed you a jigsaw puzzle and you put the pieces together. While your professional insight was invaluable, it was your personal feedback that most affirmed the work. Thank you for sharing not only what you thought, but what you felt as you waded through some very emotional material.

Thanks to Valerie Bellamy of Dog-ear Book Design. Your patience and guidance were beyond measure, especially as you watched me come full circle!

I'm grateful to those who gave such wise and generous feedback on the manuscript. To Nancy Evans Bush — your support and critical eye have been essential to this book, especially on the NDE sections. Thank you for your honesty and enthusiasm. Most of all, thank you for the vast wisdom you have given to NDE research.

To Dr. Alistair Cunningham and Dr. Rob Rutledge — your encouragement and enthusiasm are deeply appreciated. The contributions you have made to integrative care have been an inspiration to me. You are models of compassionate wisdom and holistic practice.

To Erin Montgomery, Roy Ellis, Dr. Penny Sartori, Dr. Mimi Davis, Dr. Wojciech Morzycki, my fellow chaplains and members of the psychosocial team, and to all the nurses and doctors at the QEII Health Sciences Centre, thank you for the conversations and support, not only for this book but also on the dimensions of patient care that are central to the soul. You are more than colleagues, you are my friends and mentors. It is a privilege to serve at your side.

To my good friends Scott and Gail — thank you for all your work in developing the social media platform. Scott, I'm happy to say our resolutions have been fulfilled!

To my good friends Mike and Eileen — thank you for the wine and laughter, for the campfire conversations, and for letting me know when I needed to come down to earth and speak plainly.

The individuals and families of Peace Lutheran Church were incredibly supportive throughout the years. I'm especially grateful for your prayers and comfort when I was ill. Several of you knew this book would come long before I did! All of you are part of God's story written into mine, and I am richer for it. Thank you so much.

Of course, there's no way to fully express my gratitude for the doctors and nurses who provided care to me through my own cancer journey. I literally would not be here if it were not for you. Thank you hardly seems enough.

Finally, most importantly, thank you to my family and my wife, Erika. You have been a constant source of support and encouragement. This would not have been possible without you. Erika, while I would like to promise not to be glued to the screen any more, there may yet be another book in me!

About the Author

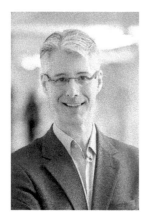

DAVID MAGINLEY, MDIV, CSCP, IS AN INTERFAITH chaplain at the QEII Health Sciences Centre in Halifax, Nova Scotia. He has survived cancer four times, which led to a profound near-death experience and explorations in consciousness and the connection of body, mind, and spirit. With degrees in philosophy and as an ordained minister, David has a deep sense of purpose in supporting others in their spiritual journey. He knows what it's like to have cancer from both sides of the hospital bed and has a sense of this life from both sides of the veil.

In addition to being an author, David is an avid photographer. His writing and images explore mortality, compassion, resilience, and hope — themes relevant to anyone seeking a deeper spiritual path, in addition to those facing cancer.

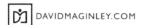 DAVIDMAGINLEY.COM

FREEMAN PATTERSON, C.M., M.DIV., R.C.A. IS AN INTERNATIONALLY REC-
ognized photographer, teacher and writer whose work explores the link
between the natural and the spiritual world. Author of over a dozen books
on photography, design, and creativity, Freeman has also written for various magazines, and been featured on CBC radio and television. For more
information, visit freemanpatterson.com.

CPSIA information can be obtained
at www.ICGtesting.com
Printed in the USA
LVHW091623200619
621865LV00005B/813/P

9 780995 881112